Fibromyalgia

Understanding
and getting relief from
pain that
won't go away

D1353204

Dr Don L. Goldenberg

Foreword by Professor Simon Wessely

PIATKUS

🍀 Visit the Piatkus website!

Piatkus publishes a wide range of bestselling fiction and non-fiction, including books on health, mind, body & spirit, sex, self-help, cookery, biography and the paranormal.

If you want to:
- read descriptions of our popular titles
- buy our books over the internet
- take advantage of our special offers
- enter our monthly competition
- learn more about your favourite Piatkus authors

VISIT OUR WEBSITE AT: www.piatkus.co.uk

Every effort has been made to ensure that the information contained in this books is complete and accurate. However, neither the publisher nor the author is engaged in rendering professional advice or services to the individual reader. The ideas, procedures, and suggestions contained in this book are not intended as a substitute for consulting with your doctor. All matters regarding your health require medical supervision. Neither the author nor the publisher shall be liable or responsible for any loss or damage allegedly arising from any information or suggestion in this book.

Copyright © 2002 by Don Goldenberg, M.D.

Consultant for UK edition: Rob Goodwin
Book design by Tiffany Kukec

This edition first published in Great Britain in 2002 by
Judy Piatkus (Publishers) Limited, 5 Windmill Street, London W1T 2JA
e-mail: info@piatkus.co.uk

Reprinted 2003

The moral rights of the author have been asserted

A catalogue record for this book is available from the British Library

ISBN 0 7499 2306 7

This book has been printed on paper manufactured with respect for the environment using wood from managed sustainable resources

Printed and bound in Great Britain
by Biddles Ltd, Guildford and King's Lynn
www.biddles.co.uk

CONTENTS

ACKNOWLEDGMENTS

DURING the past twenty years, I have had the opportunity to work with a wonderful group of clinicians and researchers dedicated to helping people with fibromyalgia and related disorders. My closest collaborations in Boston, Massachusetts, have been with Dr. Joanne Borg-Stein, Dr. Tej Sandhu, Dr. Gail Adler, and Dr. Deborah Zucker. Most of the physicians throughout the world that I have worked with or shared ideas with are mentioned in this book. It has been a special pleasure to become great friends with Drs. Robert and Sharon Bennett from Portland, Oregon.

This book would never have been possible without the encouragement and perseverance of my literary agent, Linda Konner. My editor at Perigee Books, Sheila Curry Oakes, has sharpened the focus and organization of my thoughts. My office staff, especially Janine Beauchemin, have allowed me to have some protected time to work on this project during the past few years.

A special thanks to Ken and Hazel Dreyer for their support. My own physicians, Drs. Mike Levin and Nick Browning, were always there for me in times of need.

The thousands of patients that I have been fortunate enough to meet have been a true inspiration. Watching as they have tackled difficult problems of pain and fatigue has taught me new lessons every day.

Most importantly, my family has brought me happiness each day of my life. Wendy, Julie, Thom, Michael, and Julia are my joy. And above all, my wife, Patty, has taught me about fibromyalgia, about maintaining equanimity and humour at all times, and about the true meaning of love.

Note on the UK edition of this book
The American edition of this book has been adapted for the British market: the names of drugs and medical terms have been changed to their UK equivalents. We are indebted to Rob Goodwin for his advice on this aspect of the book.

FOREWORD

Simon Wessely, MA, BM, BCh, MSc, MD, FRCP, FRCPsych, FMedSci, is Professor in Psychological Medicine at King's College Hospital, London.

FIBROMYALGIA is one of those conditions that regularly gets short changed by our health-care system. People don't die of it. There are no simple diagnostic tests, nor obvious physical signs. Diagnosis is difficult. Psychological symptoms such as depression and anxiety are frequent, which allows the unsympathetic to dismiss it as 'psychiatric', sadly revealing more about the doctor's own prejudices than anything about fibromyalgia, yet it happens. Patients are distressed and disabled, and can take up a lot of time in a busy clinic, time the hard pressed rheumatologist can ill afford.

But to ignore the problem is to turn one's back on an important and neglected group of patients, as well as to forget why doctors went into medicine in the first place. Fibromyalgia is an important medical problem – making up a substantial proportion of all those seen in rheumatology clinics in Britain. It is a frequent problem in general practice as well, even if often not diagnosed. Granted no one dies of it, but tens of thousands suffer from it, and have their lives seriously affected. The quality of life of sufferers is comparable to, and often worse than, those with conditions such as cancer or heart disease who do not have to fight to command medical respect and health service resources.

Don Goldenberg has produced a superb book that I believe offers real hope to sufferers. He is ideally placed for the task. He is a much respected rheumatologist who has been producing high-quality research papers on the subject for over two decades. He can hold his head up high at Grand Rounds and conferences across the world. When he talks, the profession listens.

But he is more than that. As the moving preface to the book shows, he and his wife have 'been there'. His is not just the dry learning of the scientific paper and textbook, important though that is. His knowledge comes also from direct experience of what it is like to experience fibromyalgia symptoms, and how one can overcome them. Hence this book achieves a rare balance of science and compassion – mixing the research evidence with the personal experience. He is ideally placed to separate fact from fiction, as he does in each of the chapters of this book. And for pedants like me who like to read chapter and verse, it is all there in the notes.

Don Goldenberg is also well placed to span the mind–body divide that so often gets in the way of medical care and understanding. For him, the distinction between mind and body is both mistaken and unhelpful. He makes it clear that the causes of fibromyalgia lie in both brain and body, and that any successful treatment must address both with equal respect.

In my own clinical practice I am frequently at a loss to know what to recommend to my patients who want to learn more about what is wrong with them. Granted there are innumerable Web sites and Internet information – far too much, in fact, for anyone to take in, and much of it is distinctly dubious. Now at last I have something that I can recommend with confidence – something that is able to stick to the scientific facts, and to separate out the truths from the fiction – but something that also speaks directly to patients. It is a pleasure to recommend this book. I hope those who read it find it helps them – and I feel confident it will.

Simon Wessely, 2002

PREFACE

UNTIL twenty years ago, fibromyalgia was an obscure medical condition – a relative curiosity, rarely mentioned at academic medical centres. While there were no books for the public written on fibromyalgia until about ten years ago, fibromyalgia, and the closely related chronic fatigue syndrome, have recently become hot topics. Magazines, newspapers, television stories, and popular books have stimulated widespread interest. However, this new interest has sparked confusion and controversy about fibromyalgia. Hype and misinformation have been more prevalent than facts and rational advice. People with fibromyalgia have been bombarded with quick fixes, pseudoscientific claims, and misguided zeal. I am concerned with the half-truths surrounding fibromyalgia. Despite the coverage it has received recently in the media, I recognize that we have a long way to go before we grasp the many facets of this perplexing disorder. Writing this book allows me to set the record straight.

During the past twenty years, I have dedicated much of my career to the illness called fibromyalgia. This commitment stemmed from my wife's struggle with fibromyalgia, which began in 1977. Together, Patty and I learned to deal effectively with this very common and perplexing condition. In my medical practice, I have established a comprehensive team approach to help patients achieve improved health in mind and body.

Fibromyalgia has taught me two valuable lessons. I now appreciate that many of the symptoms that cause human suffering are not easily categorized and don't fit neatly within a single disease. Doctors are trained to evaluate a patient's symptoms. The word *symptom*, as derived from Greek *symptōma,* translates to 'anything that has befallen one.' Common problems such as chronic pain and chronic fatigue are often not caused by an organic disease. Fibromyalgia's symptoms include chronic pain and exhaustion. Although these symptoms cause illness and suffering, no definite structural or biological abnormalities have been found. There is no demonstrable disease that indicates that fibromyalgia is a psychological disorder. Such assumptions are based on the archaic division of the mind from the body. Fibromyalgia has taught me that new illness models are needed if we are to better understand and treat chronic pain, exhaustion, and headaches.

The other important lesson that I have learned is that fibromyalgia affects each person differently. Hippocrates taught 'study the patient rather than the disease.' To illustrate the wide range of experiences of fibromyalgia, in the following chapters I will share my wife's story as well as the stories of some of my patients. I believe that, in order to understand fibromyalgia, or any illness, we need to understand ourselves.

Following that logic, I should reveal something about myself. The emotional as well as the physical aspects of illness have always intrigued me. This started when my parents had the foresight to send me to Dr. Kaufman, a psychiatrist, when I was ten. As with many children, emotional distress resulted in my overeating and becoming withdrawn and unhappy. I don't remember much about those therapeutic sessions, but because of them I became a happier, healthier child. I decided then and there that I wanted to be a physician, possibly a psychiatrist. I wanted to help people in the way that Dr. Kaufman had helped me. Eventually I decided to become a rheumatologist, a field which provided me with great flexibility in treating people with chronic illness.

During my adolescence, I became fascinated with the dynamic roles that nature and nurture have in shaping our lives. My mother was strong-willed, self-sufficient, and introverted. I admired these traits as she battled with breast cancer and bacterial endocarditis during my teens. My dad was a professional football player with the Green Bay Packers from 1933 to 1945. He was outgoing, open, and very comfortable being the centre of attention. Praise from his friends and fans nourished his zest for life. He would take me along on his many speaking engagements, where his football and professional wrestling stories fascinated young and old alike. My comfort level being in front of audiences began at an early age.

As an adult I experienced a number of chronic illnesses. Each has modified my thinking about fibromyalgia. As a junior doctor in 1969, I experienced a mono-like illness that left me exhausted for three months. Over the next thirty years, I have had recurrent bouts of unexplained fatigue. In 1993 I began having daily headaches. I had had occasional migraine headaches for years so I wasn't too concerned at first. But eventually these headaches became intolerable. I spent hours trying to figure out the cause. I tinkered with my diet. Was I not sleeping enough, not getting enough exercise? I started to worry about fumes in the hospital and the ventilation in my office.

I kept telling myself – I can handle this. If anyone knew how to deal with medical uncertainty, it was me. This is what I was trained to do. As a rheumatologist (an arthritis specialist), the specific cause of most conditions that I treat is obscure. Therapy is usually palliative, easing symptoms but seldom curative. Much of my research had been devoted to understanding the role of uncertainty in illness outcomes. Now I had lost perspective, the very thing I warned my patients about.

So, like most of my patients, I began to 'doctor shop.' In short order, I consulted with a specialist in internal medicine, an ear-nose-and-throat specialist, an allergist, an ophthalmologist, and a neurologist. I, just like most patients, wanted to find scientific or medical explanations for my illness. As doctors we are taught that an accurate disease diagnosis must be established for treatment to be effective. How could I get better if I didn't know what was wrong? My headaches did not respond to migraine remedies, pain medications, muscle relaxants, or anti-inflammatory drugs. During the next few years I underwent sinus surgery twice and eventually had surgery on my skull to cure a bone infection. The headaches persisted. Feelings of despair, anger, and fear dominated my days and kept me awake at night.

I became anxious and depressed. My family doctor suggested that I see a psychiatrist. Because that had been helpful when I was a child, I agreed that it was worth trying again. Although I was convinced that my headaches were purely physical in nature, I began to feel better with counselling and antidepressant medications. This first-hand experience made me more attuned to the emotional component of chronic illness. Eventually, I discovered better ways to handle stress and learned to be more flexible. My compassion for people's suffering was broadened.

Early in my medical career, I was not interested in ill-defined illnesses such as fibromyalgia or chronic fatigue syndrome. My training and interests focused on the systemic, immune diseases such as rheumatoid arthritis and systemic lupus erythematosus. This all changed when Patty began suffering from unexplained aches and pains all over her body. Her struggle with fibromyalgia opened my eyes to its many faces.

1

What Is Fibromyalgia?

PATTY and I met during her first year at the University of Wisconsin. She grew up in Long Island, New York – the 'all-American' girl. Secretary of the student council, a member of the tennis, field hockey, and cheerleading squads, she was smart, pretty, and popular. When we first met, I was blown away by her confidence, charm, and energy. Always upbeat and smiling, Patty had a good word for everybody. We were perfectly balanced. I saw the glass half or nearly empty, whereas Patty saw it half full.

We fell in love and got married just as I started medical school. Our two children followed while I was in medical school and during my training as a junior doctor. Later, many of our family activities revolved around the sports we did together. Patty taught me to ski, and skiing trips to the American West or to Europe became a yearly pilgrimage. We took dance and golf lessons together. Patty is a natural athlete. Whether dancing, swimming, skiing, or playing golf, everything she does is graceful. I struggle with these endeavours and have always envied the way Patty makes them look so easy.

After completing my internal medicine training, I decided to specialize in rheumatology. This was a field that would satisfy my interest in the long-term management of chronic illness. It was a dynamic field with new and exciting discoveries being made about the immunological aspects of the rheumatic diseases. I was fortunate to be accepted into one of the premier rheumatology training programmes, located in Boston, Massachusetts, where I would have access to the newest information and discoveries. Our family fell in love with New England and decided to spend the rest of our lives in the Boston area. Before we could settle down, however, I had a two-year obligation to the army, and we were stationed in the Pacific Northwest. Afterwards, I joined the faculty at Boston University Medical Center and we moved back to Boston. During the first ten years of our marriage we moved seven different times. No matter where we moved to or how long we stayed, Patty smoothed out each transition. Wherever we went, new friends would seek out her advice and comfort.

Things were going well in our first real home back in Boston when suddenly, in 1977, Patty's boundless energy faded. Intense aches and pains spread over her muscles and joints. Pounding headaches became a daily occurrence. Every day she awoke feeling exhausted, but a specialist in internal medicine could find nothing abnormal. I began to wonder whether she was simply worn out. The moves with two small children must have been taking a toll. My work made it difficult to be around enough to help out.

Patty and I consulted the best specialists in Boston. Nothing was detected. I kept waiting for someone to come up with a diagnosis, but test after test came back negative. A number of anti-inflammatory and pain-relieving drugs were tried, but to no avail.

Patty's description of fibromyalgia heralded what thousands of patients would report to me during the next two decades: *I feel bruised all over. Every part of my body hurts. My bones ache. My neck and shoulders are so stiff that I can't turn my head. It hurts to take a deep breath. My legs throb and are either numb or are burning. Even my skin feels sore and sensitive. Every time I try to exercise, I am totally exhausted. A walk around the block is a struggle. It feels like I'm stuck in heavy mud. I wake up feeling like I haven't slept at all. I'm so tired that I can't concentrate. My eyes have become so dry that they feel like sandpaper. My mouth feels like it is stuffed with cotton wool.*

When you are constantly sick, but doctors find nothing wrong, you either fear the worst or question your own sanity. Initially, Patty and I worried that some life-threatening disease like multiple sclerosis or lupus would emerge. As three years passed and the medical tests were still negative, we both began to wonder if her symptoms were psychological. Patty asked me, *Do you think this could all be in my head?* Patty's mother and sister had both suffered bouts of depression, and she was well aware of the hereditary basis of mood disturbances.

During the summer of 1980, we drove down to visit friends in Alabama. Patty was looking forward to the trip and planned it down to the last detail. By the time we reached our friends, Patty was so exhausted she could barely function. Yet she never complained, always smiling in front of our kids and friends. During the trip home, she slept for hours on end. Her nausea was so bad that she began to dread going to restaurants. Her face lost its healthy glow. When we returned home, Patty reiterated her concern that her symptoms were caused by depression:

This pain is wearing me out. I have had so many tests and seen so many doctors and no one can figure this out. Maybe it is all in my head after all. I'm certainly now getting depressed over all of this. There seems to be no end to it.

We held each other. I felt so helpless. Three years of suffering had gone by. Patty had been poked and probed by all kinds of specialists, but no diagnosis had been made. I didn't know how to help her. The next day, as if in answer to our prayers, I stumbled upon a medical paper about fibromyalgia. I had heard of fibromyalgia before, but I had not paid much attention to it. My medical school professors dismissed it as a 'dustbin diagnosis,' not a specific disorder. 'Fibromyalgia' was a name used when people hurt everywhere, but nothing was really wrong. It was implied that such people were hypochondriacs.

The symptoms described in the fibromyalgia patients matched Patty's. They affected mainly women, between the ages of thirty and sixty, and involved widespread muscle and joint pain. No arthritis or systemic diseases had been found. Their blood tests and X-rays had been normal. Each patient also reported fatigue, sleep disturbances, headaches, and irritable bowel. The examination of these patients was unremarkable other than for multiple, tender points. These were located at specific sites where the muscle inserted into the bone. The tender points were found on both the right and left sides of the body.

Carefully following the technique described in the medical report, I examined Patty for these tender points. I applied about nine pounds of pressure, enough to whiten my fingernail, to each point (see Figure of tender points, page 5). This began with a site next to the bony protuberance of the elbow, the so-called tennis elbow location. Patty winced in pain. I moved up to the shoulder and located the middle of the trapezius muscle, then to the sternocleidomastoid muscle that wraps around the neck. Once again, modest amounts of pressure with my finger elicited severe discomfort. Patty was extremely tender at the junction of the second rib to the sternum, a location corresponding to what is often called costochondritis. Working downwards, I pressed firmly on points at the middle and lower back, then the outer aspects of the hips and finally the inner bursa of the knees. Patty reacted with an alarming degree of pain at each site. She had every one of the typical fibromyalgia tender points. That was the first of at least twenty thousand tender point examinations that I have done during the past twenty years.

Patty and I began to read everything that we could about fibromyalgia. It didn't take long to realize that we had finally found her elusive diagnosis. Our joy at arriving at a diagnosis was tempered by the lack of information about fibromyalgia. No one seemed to know what was causing it or how to treat it effectively.

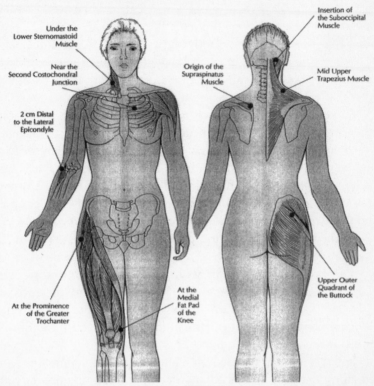

FIGURE 1. Tenderness at characteristic musculoskeletal locations establishes fibromyalgia as a consistent entity. The nine 'tender points' depicted are important in diagnosis: each is bilateral, for a total of 18 test sites widely distributed on the body surface, and tenderness on digital palpation of at least 11 in a patient with at least a three-month history of diffuse musculoskeletal pain is recommended as the diagnostic standard for fibromyalgia.

Fibromyalgia is not a new illness. Its origins, names, and explanations have gone through numerous modifications and alterations during the past century. In the mid- 1800s, doctors disentangled the symptoms of joint rheumatism (arthritis) from those of muscular rheumatism (fibromyalgia). Description of this muscular rheumatism included 'a pulling, tearing, shooting sensation with stiffness and immobility of the affected parts.' Tender points and trigger points were skillfully described in 1841 by François Valleix, who stated: 'If, in the interval of the shooting pains, one asks a patient what is the seat of his pain, he replies then by designating limited points. It is only with the aid of pressure that one discovers exactly the extent of the painful points. They are found placed in four principal points of the trajectory of different nerves. It is not very rare to encounter points painful to pressure without spontaneous pain and reciprocally.'

There was confusion, which persists to this day, about whether the pain had a muscular or a neurological origin. Valleix concluded '. . . pain, the capital symptom of neuralgia, expresses itself in different ways. If it remains concentrated in the nerves, one finds characteristic, isolated, painful points. This is neuralgia in the proper sense. If the pain spreads into the muscles, the muscular contractions are principally painful. This is muscular rheumatism.'

At the turn of the century, doctors favoured the view that the pain and tender points were caused by tissue inflammation. A famous British physician, Sir William Gowers, in his lecture *Lumbago: Its Lessons and Analogs,* coined the term 'fibrositis' in 1904. In that same year, a pathologist from Edinburgh, Dr. Ralph Stockman, reported that inflammation was present in the fibrous attachments of muscle to bone.

Initial treatment focused on eliminating the inflammation and tissue nodules as described by Stockman '. . . inflamed circumscribed parts, which are tender, painful on pressure, and if large, can be easily felt. These indurations assume various forms varying in size from a small shot or split pea to an almond, or even half a walnut. Very frequently the thickening takes the form of a strand or cord running through the fascia or subcutaneous fat.' Doctors as well as lay therapists had been practising massage for centuries and claimed that these palpable nodules were the source of pain. It made sense to manipulate or massage them away.

To this day, doctors tell patients that muscle nodules cause the pain in fibromyalgia. There has never been good evidence for this conclusion. Even a century ago experts postulated that the nervous system, rather than the muscles, was responsible for the pain. Sir William Osler, the father of modern-day medicine, reported in 1909 that muscular rheumatism was common but, '. . . it is by no means certain that the muscular tissues are the site of the disease.' Drs. Lewis and Kellgren demonstrated that muscle pain follows patterns consistent with neurological pain. They reproduced the symptoms of fibromyalgia by injecting saline into specific muscle sites. The subsequent pain, numbness, and burning spread down the muscle in characteristic patterns. The numbness and tingling sensations are referred to as 'paresthesias' and the term 'trigger point' was coined. The analogy was that pressure on these points would be the stimulus for symptoms, just as pulling a trigger fires a bullet down the barrel of a gun.

Physicians such as Michael Good in England, Michael Kelly in Australia, and Janet Travell in the United States, kept the notion of trigger points alive. Terms such as 'fibrositis,' 'muscular rheumatism,' 'myofibrositis,' 'myofasciitis,' and 'myofascial pain' were used interchangeably. Inflammatory or metabolic abnormalities of the muscle were postulated. Trigger points were also said to induce such diverse symptoms as nausea, vomiting, abdominal cramps, diarrhoea, dizziness, and visual disturbances. However, mainstream medicine rejected the notion that trigger points represented specific pathology. Muscles were biopsied and carefully examined, but no tissue inflammation was found.

Gradually, scientifically based medical journals and textbooks began to focus on the psyche in chronic muscle pain. The most prestigious rheumatology textbooks in the United States and England placed fibromyalgia or fibrositis in their chapters under the heading *psychogenic rheumatism*. Fibromyalgia was caught in the mind–body debate.

In the early 1980s, a number of rheumatologists in the United States began to share their experiences with this illness. A small fraternity of these doctors, including myself, Rob Bennett, Fred Wolfe, Jon Russell, and Muhammed Yunus, began to publish our observations. We became proficient at performing a tender point examination and used it to confirm the diagnosis of fibromyalgia. We became aware of the associated symptoms such as fatigue, sleep disturbances, headaches, bowel irritability, and mood disturbances. I focused much of my early research on these associations.

A large database was established and we collected a vast amount of medical information on patients with fibromyalgia. We contrasted the symptoms and the laboratory and physical examinations of these patients with those of healthy, age- and sex-matched people, as well as making comparisons with other rheumatic complaints.

A number of us met for a brainstorming session at the home of Dr. Frederick Wolfe in Wichita, Kansas. Our goal was to determine if a simple set of symptoms and physical findings could help doctors diagnose fibromyalgia and could differentiate fibromyalgia from other painful disorders. Fred Wolfe was chosen to organize the meeting and to collate the large amount of data that each centre had gathered during the prior two years. Wolfe was uniquely qualified to do this. He had been instrumental in sorting out the important epidemiological and clinical features of many rheumatic disorders. Remarkably, he does this research while keeping up his solo rheumatology practice. Fred took advantage of computer-generated medical information well ahead of others. He did it without the help of the biostatisticians and epidemiologists that populate major medical centres.

For the next few days we scanned the material from the fibromyalgia database. With the help of a computer-generated analysis, we reached a consensus on the most important diagnostic criteria. Eventually, these were adopted as the 1990 American College of Rheumatology Classification Criteria for the diagnosis of fibromyalgia. These criteria have allowed investigators throughout the world to approach the diagnosis of fibromyalgia with much greater consistency. If I enrol a fibromyalgia patient in a study in Boston, a rheumatologist from Australia or Germany will be familiar with the clinical characteristics of that patient. The criteria were also instrumental in promoting awareness and acceptance of fibromyalgia in the medical community.

Fibromyalgia has undoubtedly caused chronic, unexplained

pain in millions of people during the past century, but simply had not been recognized as a discrete illness. Dr. Juan Canoso and his associate Dr. Martinez-Lavin surmised that the painter Frida Kahlo had fibromyalgia. In 1925, when Kahlo was eighteen, a severe accident resulted in multiple fractures and prolonged immobilization. The rest of her life was dominated by severe, widespread pain and profound fatigue. Many diagnoses were excluded and several surgical procedures were done on her spine. None was helpful. Doctors Martinez-Lavin and Canoso wrote '. . . during periods of immobilization in a plaster corset, she used a special easel, and a mirror was attached to the canopy of her bed so that she could focus on herself. . . . A drawing in Frida's diary depicts herself in pain and eleven arrows point to anatomic sites that are near the conventional fibromyalgia tender points. Of course, because fibromyalgia is an illness without anatomic seque-lae, our contention cannot be proven or disproven. What appears certain is that Frida's self-portraits convey widespread pain and anguish with the emotional overtones that fibromyalgia patients frequently use to describe their illness.'

Fibromyalgia is present everywhere in the world, though the prevalence varies from study to study and country to country. In the United States and Canada, fibromyalgia has been found in 3 to 5 percent of women and 1 to 2 percent of men. At ages 60 to 70, 7 percent of all women have symptoms of fibromyalgia. This works out to six to ten million people with fibromyalgia in the United States alone. The prevalence from other countries such as England, Australia, Netherlands, Sweden, Norway, Germany, Italy, Israel, and Mexico is comparable.

Fibromyalgia most often occurs in previously healthy people. Of people with fibromyalgia, 50 percent attribute the onset of their symptoms to an injury, an infection, stress, or emotional trauma. The others don't know how it began. Some people have had symp-toms as long as they can remember. Fibromyalgia occurs in about 20 percent of people after a serious neck injury. It commonly follows Lyme disease or infection with the hepatitis virus. Any age group can be affected. In one report, 6 percent of all children had fibromyalgia. At every age, women with fibromyalgia outnumber men by eight to one. Fibromyalgia is more common in people who have rheumatic disorders or inflammatory diseases than in the normal population. Between 10–40 percent of people with systemic lupus erythematosus and rheumatoid arthritis have fibromyalgia.

Now that fibromyalgia has been characterized and defined, research can focus on understanding its mechanisms. Patty and I have gradually come to recognize that the muscle pain is not related to tissue damage. The most important misconception about the disorder is that fibromyalgia is a disease of muscle inflammation or biochemical defects. Studies by many investigators throughout the world have concluded that the structure and chemical constituents of the muscles, ligaments, tendons, and joints in fibromyalgia are normal. However, there are some subtle alterations of muscle function. For example, the muscles do not relax normally between contractions, which results in muscle fatigue. These changes may be related to lack of fitness and inactivity. Fortunately, no permanent muscle damage occurs.

That is good news because fibromyalgia, in contrast to arthritis or degenerative nerve disease, causes no progressive degeneration or deterioration. But, if there is no inflammation or deterioration, why does it hurt so much?

The truth is, we don't know. Those who tell you that they know what causes fibromyalgia are probably trying to sell you something. No single cause of fibromyalgia has been found. Many physical, biological, and environmental factors contribute to fibromyalgia. The eight to one female-to-male ratio in fibromyalgia suggests that hormones such as oestrogen are involved. Strengthening that hypothesis, we have found that many women experience more pain with each menstrual cycle. Similar exacerbations are common with migraine, termed menstrual migraine. About 50 percent of women with fibromyalgia report that their symptoms remit during pregnancy. However, there is no evidence for oestrogen excess or deficiency in fibromyalgia. There are also gender differences in pain sensitivity, which may be related to sex hormones. Females of all species, humans, monkeys, fish, and birds, are more sensitive to painful stimuli than their male counterparts. Fibromyalgia is more common in women with elevated prolactin levels. Fibromyalgia has been induced by the administration of gonadotropin-releasing hormone used to treat endometriosis. Some of the gender differences may be tied in with changes in the hypothalamic-pituitary-adrenal axis. Recent reports have linked hyposecretion of cortisol, serotonin, and other neurohormones to low serum androgen levels in fibromyalgia. However, the exact relationship of fibromyalgia with different female hormones is still uncertain.

There is also a genetic predisposition to fibromyalgia. If a member of your family has fibromyalgia, the chances of you getting fibromyalgia are two or three times greater than in the general population. Preliminary research has detected that certain serotonin receptor genes are more common in fibromyalgia patients compared with the general population.

During the past twenty years, fibromyalgia research has focused on the nervous system. Patty and I were intrigued by the 1975 findings of Dr. Harvey Moldofsky demonstrating that sleep is not restorative in people with fibromyalgia. Dr. Moldofsky is a psychiatrist and world-famous expert in sleep disorders. He began studying the sleep patterns of patients with fibromyalgia while working with a Canadian rheumatologist, Dr. Hugh Smythe. I attended a number of meetings with Dr. Moldofsky and became very impressed with his work. Subsequently, I visited him at his hospital and home in Toronto, Canada. Trying to unravel the mysteries of fibromyalgia has afforded me the chance to work with a diverse group of scientists. Dr. Moldofsky was the first of numerous psychiatrists, sleep experts, endocrinologists, and rehabilitation specialists with whom I collaborated.

Patty was keenly aware that her pain and fatigue correlated closely with the quality of her sleep. She had never experienced sleep disturbances before. She fell asleep quickly, but her sleep was no longer refreshing. Patty said: *I sleep so lightly that I can hear a pin drop. Every little noise wakes me. Whenever I roll over, the pain in my back or hips wakes me up. It feels like a truck ran me over in the morning, no matter how long I stay in bed.*

Sleep abnormalities are very common in fibromyalgia as well as in chronic fatigue syndrome (CFS), headaches, chronic back pain, and depression. Dr. Moldofsky was the first to demonstrate that so-called stage 4 (deep, non-dream) sleep is fragmented in fibromyalgia. He also experimentally induced these sleep disturbances in healthy people by waking them whenever their brain wave pattern indicated stage 4 sleep. Within a few days, these sleep-deprived volunteers developed the muscle pain and tender points of fibromyalgia. During stage 4 sleep our bodies recover from the stresses of daily life. A potent immune modulator, interleukin, as well as growth hormone, are secreted largely during stage 4 sleep. Lack of stage 4 sleep causes us to feel fatigued, our muscles get sore, and we are less able to combat infections.

After talking to Dr. Moldofsky, I started Patty on 20 mg of amitriptyline at bedtime. Within two days her sleep and energy improved dramatically. Medications including tricyclic antidepressants, such as amitriptyline, help restore stage 4 sleep and have been helpful in fibromyalgia. Patty has taken small amounts of amitriptyline at bedtime for twenty years with minimal side effects – occasionally dry mouth or constipation. These drugs also decrease pain and relax muscles. Amitriptyline has been used to treat headaches, other forms of chronic pain, and irritable bowel syndrome (IBS). Patty also takes aspirin or nonsteroidal anti-inflammatory medications (NSAIDs) to decrease the muscle pain. At certain times, she has taken small amounts of the newer selective serotonin reuptake inhibitor antidepressants (SSRIs), such as fluoxetine (Prozac) or paroxetine (Seroxat), which have helped improve her energy.

Patty's response to antidepressant medication provided more evidence that the central nervous system was important to understanding fibromyalgia. Investigations into abnormal sleep and the therapeutic efficacy of antidepressants got scientists interested in the role of neurohormones in fibromyalgia. My own research, including my colleague Dr. Gail Adler at the Harvard Medical School, has explored the role of the hypothalamic-pituitary-adrenal (HPA) axis, the stress axis, in fibromyalgia.

The brain's hormonal response to stress involves complicated pathways. One of the central hormones, called 'cortisol releasing hormone' or CRH, can be thought of as a thermostat regulating the release of substances such as adrenal-cortical-releasing hormone (ACTH), cortisol, and catecholamines such as adrenaline and nor-adrenaline. Many of the symptoms in fibromyalgia are similar to the physiological effects experienced when people are withdrawn from these glucocorticoid hormones. This steroid withdrawl situation causes fatigue, joint pain, muscle pain, sleep disturbances, cognitive disturbances, and gastrointestinal complaints. It is logical to think that many of the symptoms involved in fibromyalgia and CFS could be related to alterations of this stress-activated hormonal system.

Dr. Adler put fifteen of my fibromyalgia patients through a complicated series of experiments to check the status of their HPA axis. Adler found that they had a weaker response of their stress axis compared with healthy controls. Dr. Leslie Crofford at the University of Michigan Medical School has published similar results. A relatively sluggish CRH response after stress is an important part of the fibromyalgia puzzle.

Another altered hormone in fibromyalgia patients is growth hormone. This hormone is important in muscle function and is largely produced during deep sleep. Dr. Robert Bennett and co-workers demonstrated that people with fibromyalgia have lower growth-hormone levels than healthy people. When fibromyalgia patients with the lowest growth-hormone levels were given sup-plementary growth hormone, many of their fibromyalgia symp-toms improved. Dr. Russell and Dr. Yunus have investigated the role of serotonin and other neurotransmitters in fibromyalgia. Dr. Dan Clauw and Dr. Martinez-Lavin have led the way in studies of the role of the autonomic nervous system in fibromyalgia.

We still have a long way to go before we can translate these phys-iological abnormalities into more specific treatments for pain and fatigue. Currently, medications used in fibromyalgia are largely employed by trial and error. A few randomized, controlled, placebo-based trials have documented that drugs such as amitriptyline and fluoxetine are more effective than placebo, but treatment must be individualized. Medications are only one part of a comprehensive treatment plan that will be described in later chapters.

As soon as Patty's sleep was restored her energy returned. Then she resumed her regular cardiovascular exercise. People with fibromyalgia need to keep as active as possible. It may seem counter-intuitive, but exercise will help break the pain cycle. Pain causes muscle spasm. Spasm interferes with oxygen flow to the muscle. Low levels of oxygen lead to lactic acid accumulation in muscle, causing more pain. I advise my patients to do regular cardiovascular exercise, which will enhance muscle oxygen supply, and to stretch their muscles, which will diminish spasm.

Exercise came naturally to Patty. She now feels better when she walks or runs or does an aerobics class. I was so proud of her when she completed the Boston Marathon five years ago. Not everyone will be able to run marathons, but everyone with chronic illness can exercise and be more active.

Patty recalls: *Before knowing what was wrong, I was afraid to exercise, thinking that it would hurt my muscles even more. Once I began to exercise regularly, I felt human again. Small amounts of amitriptyline at night gave me the first decent night's sleep that I'd had in years. I now do everything that I want although I have learned to pace myself. Every once in a while, fibromyalgia hits me hard again. Especially when I become too complacent about it. But I know what to do to help and I can ride out the down times without worrying that there will be nothing but bad times ahead. A few years ago, I even ran the Boston Marathon. I finished far back, but I finished. Struggling with fibromyalgia was very much like training for a marathon. Taking one step at a time, slowly, but always moving forwards, worked for me.*

Patty's illness made me acutely aware of the suffering that fibromyalgia may cause. I am proud to be one of the researchers who brought fibromyalgia into the medical mainstream. At the same time, I am humbled to admit that it took my own wife's illness to make me appreciate the profound impact of ill-defined disorders such as fibromyalgia and CFS.

FICTION

- Fibromyalgia is a new illness.

- It is a disease of muscle.

- There are no physiological abnormalities in fibromyalgia.

- There is no effective treatment.

- It lasts forever.

FACTS

- 'Fibromyalgia' is the name applied to a group of common symptoms that were well described more than a century ago. These symptoms include chronic, generalized muscle pain, fatigue, sleep disturbances, headaches, and irritable bowel.

- Characteristic tender points where muscles attach to bones are the only helpful physical finding in fibromyalgia. These points do not represent muscle inflammation or structural damage.

- Changes in central nervous system hormones that regulate sleep, pain, and energy are important in this illness.

- Treatment includes medications that decrease pain and improve sleep and non-medicinal physical therapies and exercise.

- Fibromyalgia usually improves with treatment and may gradually disappear.

2

Why Is the Diagnosis So Difficult and So Controversial?

PATTY's illness focused my clinical and research attention on fibromyalgia. In 1987, the prestigious medical journal *JAMA* (*Journal of the American Medical Association*) published my review of fibromyalgia. Its title, 'Fibromyalgia: An Emerging but Controversial Condition,' turned out to be prophetic. Fibromyalgia is now widely accepted as a common illness. However, everything about fibromyalgia is still controversial. On 13 November, 2000, in *The New Yorker,* Dr. Jerry Groopman stated: 'In fact, fibromyalgia has become such a contentious medical topic that most of the doctors I spoke with specified that their views were off the record. Some feared that any hint of sympathy would cause a deluge of referrals; others worried that voicing skepticism about the syndrome would make them vulnerable to public attack.'

Even the name 'fibromyalgia' has been challenged. It was selected because it describes the two cardinal features of the syndrome, 'myalgia' or widespread muscle pain and 'fibro' to indicate the tenderness where the 'fibrous' muscle tissue attaches to bone. This new nomenclature avoids any reference to tissue inflammation, in contrast to fibrositis. Critics comment that the name 'fibromyalgia' suggests that this is a muscle disease despite research demonstrating that it is not. However, there are more fundamental reasons for the controversies enveloping fibromyalgia.

Getting a diagnosis of fibromyalgia is no easy task. The symptoms of fibromyalgia are far more diverse than pain. Problems with dizziness, memory, bowel and bladder irritability, headaches, weight fluctuations, allergies, sinus and nasal congestion, hearing and vision changes, and unusual sensitivity to numerous medications, chemicals, or environmental stimuli all create diagnostic confusion.

Because so many conditions must be excluded, it may take considerable time to nail down the fibromyalgia diagnosis. Often patients and their doctors are worried that diseases such as lupus, multiple sclerosis, or cancer are being missed. Once symptoms persist for months or years in the absence of any physical or laboratory abnormalities, there is little chance that a dangerous disease is lurking, still undetected. As the patient keeps searching for a diagnosis many doctors are consulted, and more and more tests are ordered.

Patty went through hundreds of blood tests to find out what was wrong. Being a rheumatologist, I was most concerned that a rheumatic disease was brewing. Patty's eye and mouth dryness, termed sicca syndrome, and her dramatic fingertip reaction to cold, termed Raynaud's phenomenon, are common symptoms in immune diseases. They are also common in fibromyalgia. I began to worry that Patty might be developing an immunological disease, such as systemic lupus erythematosus (lupus). Lupus most often affects women between the ages of thirty and fifty. It causes joint and muscle pain and exhaustion. I sent Patty to a rheumatology colleague whom I considered to be the best diagnostician in Boston. He also suspected a disease of the connective tissues, such as lupus or scleroderma. A series of immunological blood tests were ordered.

One of these, an antinuclear antibody (ANA) test, was positive.

This heightened my worst suspicion that Patty might have lupus. The positive ANA test result meant that Patty's blood contained an antibody that reacted against her own nuclear material. Immune diseases are characterized by such antibodies. They are signs of an excessive and misguided immune system. Instead of forming antibodies to fight a foreign invader, like a virus, people with immune diseases make antibodies against themselves. The presence of such antibodies helps to confirm the diagnosis of an immune disease, provided the characteristic clinical signs and symptoms are present. Almost every patient with lupus has a positive ANA test.

Now we finally had a test that might indicate a serious disease like lupus. Yet, I knew that a positive ANA test did not mean that Patty had lupus. The presence of such antibodies is not necessarily 'pathological.' Sometimes, for no good reason, the body makes auto-antibodies such as the antinuclear antibody. Among healthy women, 5 to 10 percent have a positive ANA.

People with fibromyalgia are often found to have abnormal tests. In our technologically advanced medical system, many doctors and patients put too great a stock in 'tests.' These might include blood tests, X-rays, computer aided tomography (CAT) scans, or magnetic resonance imaging scans (MRIs). However, tests rarely make a diagnosis. Blood tests or sensitive techniques such as MRIs are most helpful when they confirm a doctor's clinical judgement.

The more medical uncertainty that shrouds an illness, the more tests that are ordered. Doctors worry about missing something. Patients insist on more tests to find out what is wrong with them. Millions of people with common yet obscure ailments such as fibromyalgia are subjected to excess investigation, misdiagnosis, and overtreatment.

Over the past twenty years, I have seen hundreds of people with isolated 'false positive' immunological blood tests. Based on such tests they were told that they probably had lupus or rheumatoid arthritis. Patients often request that I test them for lupus or multiple sclerosis. However, indiscriminate testing creates diagnostic and therapeutic uncertainties and often leads to needless worry. If enough tests are performed on a person, some will be 'abnormal' by chance alone. Doctors know that a careful history and physical examination will provide a diagnosis 90 percent of the time. Most 'tests' simply confirm the clinical diagnosis. I spend a lot of time explaining to patients why blood test 'abnormalities' do not necessarily correlate with any disease.

Patty and I began a new round of doctor shopping. Patty consulted with a neurologist because of the peculiar numbness and tingling sensations in her arms and legs, which could be caused by carpal tunnel syndrome or a herniated disc. An electromyogram and nerve-conduction study were done to see if any nerve disease was present. Electrodes were inserted up and down the nerves in Patty's arms and legs. Then tiny jolts of electricity were applied and the electrical conduction across each nerve was measured. This was not a pleasant experience. The test was normal and we went back to the drawing board. Diagnosing fibromyalgia is always difficult. Unfortunately, there is no gold standard.

There is also confusion about the specificity of syndromes like fibromyalgia. I keep reminding my patients that fibromyalgia is a label we have applied to their symptoms. The name is no more specific than the diagnosis of headaches. Fibromyalgia symptoms overlap with those of other syndromes like CFS.

Andrea, a fifty-five-year-old housewife, called me from California. She had been diagnosed with CFS four years earlier. Antibiotics, antiviral agents, vitamin therapy, and nutritional supplements had not been helpful. In addition to her fatigue, she described pain all over her body. Andrea decided to fly up to see me so that I could determine whether she 'had also acquired fibromyalgia.'

Her history and examination were consistent with fibromyalgia as well as CFS. Andrea told me that she was allergic to most medications. She had visited two different complementary medicine practitioners and had been treated with a homeopathic remedy.

Andrea was taking echinacea, nystatin, melatonin, and two different Chinese herbal ingredients. She was wearing magnets on her
back and inside the soles of her shoes.

My examination demonstrated the typical fibromyalgia tender
points. Andrea, like Patty, fitted the diagnostic criteria for both
CFS and fibromyalgia. So do most people. This isn't surprising if
one remembers that these syndromes consist of groups of symptoms. If you suffer from chronic pain you will most likely suffer
from chronic fatigue and chronic headaches.

Some doctors and patients have also argued with my assertion
that fibromyalgia and CFS are essentially one and the same. They
point to studies suggesting differences in certain hormones. Subtle
immune alterations have been commonly noted in CFS, but all
studies have demonstrated marked clinical, epidemiological, and
biological overlap of fibromyalgia and CFS. At this stage, the
only absolute conclusions that clinicians agree upon is that each of
these syndromes is common, has no clear cause, and has many
overlapping features.

The main reason why fibromyalgia is so controversial is
because there is nothing much to see or measure. The physical
examination and laboratory tests don't demonstrate consistent
abnormalities. There is no known cause, and no cure. This has led
to serious concerns about the diagnosis of fibromyalgia. 'Real'
medical disorders have 'objective' evidence of illness. Objective
data are irrefutable. Subjective symptoms are tied to a particular
person's perspective. They are 'subject' to that person's bias.
When there are no objective measures of disease present, the doctor must take the patient's word. Doctors question whether a person with only subjective complaints is 'really' sick. An artificial
hierarchy of suffering has emerged. People with diseases like cancer or rheumatoid arthritis are thought to be suffering legiti-
mately. Conditions like fibromyalgia are thought to be
psychosomatic and not as worthy of medical attention.

Critics comment that pain, fatigue, bowel disturbances, insomnia, depression, and anxiety are experienced by every human

being. Why should those universal symptoms be referred to as a specific illness? Doctors relegate symptoms without disease to second-class status. My mentors advised me that studying fibromyalgia was not 'real' science. My research would never get funded in such a 'soft' field. My career advancement would be stymied.

This line of reasoning demeans illnesses like fibromyalgia or CFS. The prevailing attitude it engenders is that any person who succumbs to such complaints is weak. A prominent rheumatologist equates fibromyalgia with being 'out of sorts.' He says that we all have bad days characterized by stiffness and achiness, fatigue, loss of well-being, and preoccupation with our bowels. He claims that the diagnosis of fibromyalgia does harm because assigning a label to the normal hardships of life 'teaches people to be sick.'

A neurologist who has become a national spokesman for antifibromyalgia sentiments asserts that fibromyalgia is 'not a legitimate disease, in contrast to rheumatoid arthritis.' He proclaimed: 'Fibromyalgia is not just overdiagnosed, it downright does not exist. There is no empiricism to fibromyalgia. Just wild speculation. People with fibromyalgia do not have a specific medical disorder and they are harmed by giving them a name or treating them medically. It makes them feel crippled.'

CFS and fibromyalgia are termed 'functional syndromes,' in contrast to organic illness. For some, this means that a hodgepodge of symptoms are elevated to the status of a disease. This status results from popular discourse rather than scientific evidence. Critics of CFS and fibromyalgia point out that similar disorders come and go based on public attention and attitudes. Diagnoses such as neurasthenia, chronic brucellosis, chronic mononucleosis, benign myalgic encephalomyelitis, sick building syndrome, multiple chemical sensitivity, and chronic Epstein-Barr virus (CEBV) infection go in and out of favour. There is some truth to this argument. Society and our culture play an enormous role in the expression and acceptability of illness.

Even my friend and fibromyalgia co-investigator Fred Wolfe

now questions the wisdom of a fibromyalgia diagnosis: 'When we started out in the eighties, we saw patients going from doctor to doctor with pain. We believed that by telling them they had fibromyalgia we reduced stress and reduced medical utilization. This idea, a great, humane idea that we can interpret their distress as fibromyalgia and help them – it didn't turn out that way. My view now is that we are creating an illness rather than curing one. If you give them the diagnosis of fibromyalgia, pain is allowed to dominate their life. By receiving this diagnosis and taking medications, people become card-carrying members of the "fibromyalgia club."'

Indeed, misguided disease labels can have an untoward influence on our health. People with elevated blood pressure are told that they have hypertension. Hopefully, that diagnosis will result in appropriate medication and healthy lifestyle changes. However, if a person with an elevated blood pressure sees himself as a 'hypertensive,' as a timebomb of inexorably decaying vascular derangement, his fear, anger, and hopelessness may be overwhelming.

Explaining the illness, rather than labelling the illness, is essential. When I tell people that they have fibromyalgia, I make clear what that implies. Fibromyalgia is simply a term for common symptoms that are present throughout the population. Every human has been wracked with pain at times. Most of us have been exhausted. If such symptoms come and go, they are not perceived as specific illnesses. However, when these symptoms persist, they create distress and suffering – people become ill. Labelling persistent symptoms gives them context and allows patients to take action based on that knowledge.

Doctors are most comfortable when a diagnosis conforms to a specific disease process. But, the diagnosis of fibromyalgia resolves a mystery for the patient. It defines their experience. Where would we be if the diagnosis of depression had never been made? There are no objective disease measures for depression. We all feel depressed at times. When our depression reaches a critical level, depression is an illness. Extraordinary suffering, disability, and even death may follow. The diagnosis of depression has provided medicine with a framework, a construct to study this suffering. Major breakthroughs in understanding the mechanisms and treating the symptoms of depression have emerged.

Most illness labels are somewhat arbitrary. Take hypertension. If a person's blood pressure is higher than 90–95 percent of the population, we diagnose hypertension. Similarly, if a person's pain and fatigue are greater than 90–95 percent of the population, she has fibromyalgia. The diagnoses of depression, migraine, IBS, and CFS are each based on everyday symptoms becoming extraordinarily disturbing.

The criticism that fibromyalgia and related syndromes have no scientific basis is not true. There is no single cause. There is no organ damage. There are no deaths. This does not mean that the symptoms are not real. Such a misguided critique could be applied to any variety of chronic pain disorders, as well as to headaches, depression, CFS, and IBS. The labels that have been applied to each of these conditions are descriptive. But without the labels doctors could not have begun to elucidate these illnesses. Numerous physiological abnormalities have been found in fibromyalgia. They are quite similar to alterations found in chronic headaches, chronic fatigue, and IBS. We now recognize that most people who have one of these chronic illnesses also have another. The biological and clinical significance of these overlapping features could not have been recognized without descriptive labels applied to each of these syndromes.

Most importantly, the diagnostic label helps patients. Patty and most of my patients have found the label of fibromyalgia to be 'enabling,' not 'disabling.' A diagnosis gives people an explanation for their symptoms. Patients no longer dread the future, waiting for the explosion of some hidden disease. A diagnosis of fibromyalgia is a relief to the patient who fears lupus or multiple sclerosis. The label, the diagnosis, confers legitimacy to a person's symptoms. People become less worried that their family, doctor, or employer will accuse them of malingering. The earlier the diagnosis the better because unnecessary and costly testing is kept to a minimum. Patients who had been diagnosed with fibromyalgia were ten times less likely to be hospitalized than fibromyalgia patients who had not been diagnosed.

Doctors and patients have different perspectives on this issue. An interesting report compared the views of doctors and patients as to the value of a CFS diagnosis. Of general practitioners, 70 percent were reluctant to make a diagnosis of CFS. They felt 'constrained by the scientific uncertainty regarding the cause of CFS' and concerned that the diagnosis might become a self-fulfilling prophecy. In contrast, patients thought that the diagnosis of CFS was 'enabling' because it provided a coherent explanation for their illness. When a person suffers, that person is a patient (the Latin word for 'sufferer'). We doctors see the sufferer in terms of disease. A mismatch results when no disease is found.

Patty and I were relieved when we found that her illness had a name. We recognized that the word *fibromyalgia* was only a name used to describe a group of symptoms. The diagnostic label implied nothing about a cause or mechanism of her illness. But a diagnosis will allow investigators throughout the world to investigate these symptoms, to understand this suffering. Eventually better treatment will follow. Patty recalled: *Knowing that what I had was common and was treatable and not progressive was key to my recovery. I no longer thought that there was something being missed or that I was going crazy. Even if we didn't know why I got fibromyalgia, or exactly what fibromyalgia was, the diagnosis let me put this illness in perspective. The symptoms had a name and there were a lot of people out there with exactly the same complaints. That was very reassuring. I then was free to learn how to take control of it rather than to let it control me.*

Fibromyalgia is made up of its interrelated symptoms, its component parts. To understand fibromyalgia we need to explore each of these parts. For some people, like Patty, no one symptom dominates. For others, one particular component predominates. Most often this is pain.

FICTION

- A medical illness cannot exist without objective abnormalities.

- Fibromyalgia is a 'dustbin' term.

- Fibromyalgia is a diagnosis of exclusion.

- Fibromyalgia can be easily differentiated from other illnesses such as myofascial pain and CFS.

- A diagnosis of fibromyalgia is harmful because it makes people feel sick and leads to more disability.

FACTS

- Symptoms and signs, gathered from a careful history and physical examination, are the basis for the diagnosis of fibromyalgia and related illnesses.

- Illnesses such as fibromyalgia are appropriately called 'syndromes'; this describes a group of symptoms with no known cause or defined pathology.

- We put too much stock in tests and the latest technology. Excess testing is not helpful to diagnose fibromyalgia and may generate more worry.

- The symptoms of common illnesses such as myofascial pain and CFS overlap greatly with those of fibromyalgia and treatment is similar.

- The diagnosis of fibromyalgia is helpful; it provides people with an explanation for their symptoms and alleviates their worries.

3

Why Do I Hurt All Over?

JONATHAN was thirty-four when he first came to my office. He was referred by an orthopaedic surgeon who had been treating him for chronic back pain. Sitting hunched over in our waiting room, the chair appeared too small for his considerable bulk. His wife, Bonnie, helped support Jon as he eased out of the chair and painstakingly made his way into my office. At 6 feet, 4 inches and 240 pounds, Jon's massive frame dwarfed Bonnie's tiny stature. Yet, Bonnie was obviously the one doing the heavy lifting.

Jon grew up on a farm in rural New Hampshire. He was the oldest of seven children. His father had had a number of jobs to help finance their farm. When Jon was ten, his family sold most of their land and built a dairy restaurant that eventually went out of business. By the time he was fourteen, Jon was working every day after school in a car repair workshop. He began working full-time at age seventeen and married his high school sweetheart, Bonnie, at age nineteen. They had four children.

He recounted, *I worked hard for the past ten years just to get by. My car repair work kept me busy all week. Every Saturday, I loaded heavy machinery in the town's factory. I never missed a day of work. A few years ago we moved to a two-family house just off the interstate motorway. Everything was coming together before my back injury.*

In 1984 Jon first experienced back pain while lifting some heavy machinery during his weekend job. The local orthopaedic surgeon told Jon that he had strained his back. Jon took three months off from work and the pain improved. However, when back at work, he fell on some loose tiles and his back pain returned. The pain was centred in the middle of his lower back. Jon described a constant, dull ache that was aggravated by standing and sitting, and improved with lying down. X-ray results were normal, but an MRI demonstrated lumbar disc protrusion (a 'slipped disc').

Like Patty's false positive blood tests for lupus, Jon's MRI results were misleading. Even in people with no back pain, 50 percent will have some degree of a slipped disc or degenerative disc disease on MRI examination. Therefore extreme caution must be exercised in ordering and interpreting such tests. Jon next saw a chiropractor, who said that his sacroiliac joints were out of place and that the fourth and fifth lumbar vertebrae were out of alignment. Despite this common chiropractic diagnosis, vertebrae and sacroiliac joints virtually never slip or move. The sacroiliac joints are strong and stable and are rarely the source of back pain.

Chiropractic manipulation was not helpful. Over the next year, Jon went to three different surgeons. One orthopaedic surgeon recommended spinal surgery. Another orthopaedic consultant and a neurosurgeon cautioned Jonathan to avoid surgery. They found no neurological abnormalities and suggested physical therapy and pain medication. However, Jon still couldn't work because of the pain.

He told me, *Out of frustration, I went back to the surgeon who said an operation would help me. I was desperate. How could I take care of my family? I knew there were no guarantees, but the doctor said it would get worse if the slipped disc wasn't removed.*

Jon was willing to undergo back surgery. He was not told that the odds for a successful outcome were poor. You might think that medically sophisticated patients with back pain would not be as likely to go for surgery. Most health-care professionals understand that there is no magic bullet that can treat chronic back pain. But when pain is unremitting and a surgeon says that he can fix it, most of us will take the leap. Dr. Jerry Groopman lamented his own decision about surgery in his recent book, *Second Opinion*:

'X-rays showed no clear cause for the relapse. There were no bulging discs. I saw many consultants: rheumatologists, neurosurgeons, sports medicine doctors. . . . I was emotionally frayed and bitterly frustrated by the lack of answers. The cause of my problem had to be defined and aggressive solutions applied. I was determined to be permanently repaired.' After unsuccessful back surgery, Dr. Groopman admitted, 'I finally realized that my desperate belief in a perfect solution was a fantasy . . . I have never fully recovered from the surgery. Not a day passes when I don't fail to think of my headstrong decision because of the limits on my functioning.'

In 1986, Jonathan underwent the first of three back operations. After the first back operation, he felt less pain for about six months, but then all the pain returned. A second operation to remove scar tissue was performed in 1988. Eventually, Jon had a lumbar spinal fusion in 1990. None of these procedures substantially diminished his pain. They did worsen his ability to function.

When I first met Jonathan in 1994 he was in constant pain and very limited in his activities. He told me, *I can't do the simplest things around the house without my back acting up. I haven't worked in ten years and Bonnie now works two jobs to support us. The pain is always there even if I take pain pills every few hours. When I move or twist the wrong way, a shooting pain goes from my back to lower down. It is so painful, I can't move. About two years ago, I began having pain in other places, not just my back. At various times, my neck is tight and painful, my arms ache and my legs feel like lead. I'm getting headaches all the time. If I try to get down on the floor and play with my kids I need two people to hoist me back up. I can't even throw a football around with the kids.*

They have given me every conceivable medication and nothing has worked. I took ibuprofen and naproxen and then paracetamol with codeine and none of them made a dent in the pain. The only thing that works is oxycodone. But I hate the way it makes me feel. I can't think straight and I feel depressed when I take the oxycodone. But it's the only thing that will let me get an hour of rest. Then every time I ask for more oxycodone, because it's a narcotic, the doctors look at me like I'm a drug addict.

For eight years Jon had experienced unremitting back pain. During the last two years the pain had spread to his neck and shoulders. He now had constant pain not only in his back, but also in his legs, arms, and upper body. This widespread pain was typical of fibromyalgia. After years of suffering, he felt hopeless. He could not fall asleep until 1 or 2 A.M. and then would wake every time he rolled over. He felt angry at the medical profession for 'messing up my back forever.' None of his doctors could tell Jon why his back hadn't got better or why he was now experiencing pain everywhere in his body.

Jonathan talked slowly and with a sense of despair. He had difficulty getting up and grimaced each time he moved. Bonnie often answered my questions. It seemed as though Jon would take hours to respond to simple queries. His examination demonstrated no significant neurological abnormalities. Jon was very stiff, and the slightest movement of his neck, back, or hips caused severe pain. There was widespread spasm and numerous fibromyalgia tender points when I examined Jon's muscles. As described in Gowers's 1904 treatise on lumbago, Jon's back pain had spread to include the generalized muscle pain characteristic of fibromyalgia.

At any given time, one third of Americans have a chronic pain problem. More than 50 million Americans are partially or totally disabled by chronic pain. This costs the United States 60–80 billion dollars per year in lost productivity and medical expenses. The most pervasive chronic pain problem is back pain. Chronic neck pain is almost as common. At least three months of neck or back pain at one time is to be expected by 40 percent of us. At least one episode of prolonged, widespread generalized musculoskeletal pain, typical of fibromyalgia, can be expected by 10 percent of us.

Back pain is the most common cause of work loss in the United States. Fortunately, most back pain resolves spontaneously within a few days or weeks. Most people with low back pain never consult a doctor. Acute back pain is usually caused by a muscle 'pull' or tissue injury. It responds well to rest, gentle stretches, and simple analgesics like aspirin. However, recurrent or chronic back pain doesn't respond well to anything. It is the chief complaint of more than half of all disabled workers.

During much of the past fifty years, the medical industry has led us to believe that back pain and neck pain evolve from an injury, inflammation, or structural alterations in the spine. This implied that physical intervention would cure the problem. A generation of orthopaedic surgeons, neurosurgeons, physiotherapists, specialists in rehabilitation, chiropractors, osteopaths, and acupuncturists have been treating chronic pain with purely physical modalities. Unfortunately such treatment has not been very successful. In the vast majority of people with chronic pain, there is no structural problem in the spine. Chronic pain without a definite physical cause is labelled as idiopathic pain. Some doctors interpret idiopathic to mean 'the doctor is an idiot and the patient is pathetic.'

Very little medical interest or research has focused on understanding and managing chronic pain. A minuscule fraction of the United States' medical-research budget is spent on investigating pain. Most medical students receive no formal training in understanding or treating chronic pain. Nor is there a consistent approach to chronic pain treatment. Historically, medicine has tried to overlook pain, considering it a normal part of illness and healing. It seems that the more sophisticated our biotechnology, the more we neglect the research and treatment of pain. In this age of subspecialization, each medical discipline treats pain differently. Internal medicine specialists use drugs, orthopaedic surgeons remove 'slipped' discs (a misnomer since discs don't slip), anaesthetists try nerve blocks, neurosurgeons cut pain pathways, and psychiatrists explore emotional or stress-related issues.

Jon and Dr. Groopman were equally frustrated by their doctors' inability to determine the root of their back pain. In more than 90 percent of people with chronic back pain, the exact cause is uncertain. In the other 10 percent, a discrete lesion, such as a herniated disc, spinal stenosis, osteoporosis and vertebral fractures, or tumours of the spine can be found and fixed. But most back pain is idiopathic. Until quite recently, doctors thought that low back pain was often caused by spinal disc herniation. We now know that bulging discs are common in people with no back pain. And when a protruded disc is the cause of back pain, it resolves without surgery in 90 percent of people. Unfortunately, the 1950s and 1960s saw a large number of failed back operations for 'herniated discs' in the United States. Surgery was not a panacea for most types of back pain and was not the answer for Jonathan or for Dr. Groopman.

Indications for surgery on the spine have become better refined. Disc surgery is now usually restricted to patients with unremitting pain or with nerve damage. The vast majority of people with chronic back pain will never need surgery.

An extensive diagnostic search for the cause of back pain is often a wild-goose chase. Both patients and doctors can easily get carried away by the latest technologies. Many patients with chronic back pain insist that I order an MRI study of their back. All too often an MRI demonstrates incidental disc protrusion, but the symptoms and signs do not fit with that being the cause of the pain.

Tremendous breakthroughs in understanding the mechanisms involved in pain have occurred in the past five years. Pain originates from nerve receptors called nociceptors, found in the skin, muscle, and visceral tissues. Excitation of these, myelinated A and unmyelinated C, nerve fibres transmit pain sensation to the spinal cord. In the spinal cord, pain impulses can be turned up and down.

From the spinal cord the pain neurons ascend to reach the mid-brain, the thalamus, and up to the cerebral cortex. It is here that our past experiences, emotions, thoughts, and fears modulate our perception and response to pain. Downstream, a descending pain pathway down-regulates pain.

The mechanisms involved in our response to acute, self-limited pain are logical and make perfect sense. In acute pain, nerve pathways work efficiently to prevent tissue damage. There is an orderly series of events in our pain response designed to protect us, for example after we touch a hot stove.

Chronic pain can't be so rationally explained. It persists long after any initial insult. Days or weeks after an injury or inflammation, our brains do not turn off the pain message. Our internal pain thermostat registers hot even when tissue repair of the injury is complete. The persistent pain response becomes hard-wired in our brain. Eventually, the pain takes on a life of its own.

A dramatic example is phantom limb pain. About 50–80 percent of amputees report sensations of burning and deep pain at the site of the amputated limb. The first medical description of phantom limb pain was by Ambrose Paré, a famous sixteenth-century surgeon, who wrote, 'For the patients, long after the amputation is made, say they feel pain in the amputated part. Of this they complain strongly, a thing worthy of wonder and almost incredible to people who have not experienced this.' One of the most famous characters of fiction, Captain Ahab in *Moby Dick,* was afflicted by the 'ghost' of phantom limb pain. Silas Weir Mitchell, a neurologist during the American Civil War, described many soldiers with phantom limb pain in 1871. Like the amputees with phantom limb or the person with idiopathic back pain, the pain in fibromyalgia originates in the nervous system.

One of the neurologists who is opposed to the term 'fibromyalgia' has criticized my likening of the pain mechanisms that occur in fibromyalgia to those postulated for the phantom limb syndrome. He stated '. . . with the phantom limb, you have a real lesion – the limb has been cut off! Nerves and muscle and bone are damaged.

People with fibromyalgia have intact limbs and no evidence of pathology like severed tissues.' In fact, the phantom limb pain persists even if peripheral nerve input is blocked by local anaesthetics or surgery. After the limb is amputated, there is no persistent tissue trauma to explain the months or years of pain that occurs. Rather, the nervous system has gone awry. Thus, the analogy is apt.

Phantom limb syndrome is a striking example of how dramatically the wiring of pain messages in the nervous system can go wrong. In many chronic pain conditions, nerves that normally do not transmit pain become activated to do exactly that. This is often referred to as central sensitization. With chronic painful stimuli, an avalanche of pain messages bombard the brain. Restructuring of neurons and their fibres, often termed neuroplasticity, leads to chaotic explosions of unintended pain messages.

Central sensitization of pain does not necessarily require such terrible trauma as an amputated limb. Similar sensory cortical reorganization has been demonstrated in low back pain such as Jon's. I have treated many patients who have developed chronic pain involving an arm or leg after a modest injury or immobilization. There has been no adequate explanation anatomically for the pain. The pain is associated with extreme sensitivity to touch as well as unusual cold or heat sensations. This is often termed reflex sympathetic dystrophy or complex regional pain syndrome.

In these situations, ongoing tissue injury or inflammation is not present. There may be initial tissue damage, certainly the case for the amputee with phantom limb syndrome, and Jon's back pain undoubtedly had a structural basis initially. Many people with fibromyalgia report that their pain began with trauma to their head and neck, but over time the pain spread throughout the rest of their body. The central sensitization then sets in. The pain messages become supercharged, both in the spinal cord and in the brain, and nerve fibres not previously transmitting pain messages are recruited and the pain snowballs.

Like most rheumatologists, I have never thought of myself as a pain specialist. My training in immunology and clinical rheumatology did not address the scientific basis of chronic pain. However, any investigator interested in fibromyalgia or chronic back pain must explore the mechanisms involved in pain. Rheumatologists have now begun to work with physiologists and psychologists who have been delving into the mechanisms of pain for years.

The tender points represent alterations in pain perception, not in tissue structure. The most common tender points such as over the lateral epicondyle of the elbow, the tennis elbow location, are sites that take a lot of wear and tear (see Figure 1, page 5). People with fibromyalgia are more tender than healthy people no matter which part of their body is palpated. This fits with the notion that the primary pain factor is in the central nervous system rather than the musculoskeletal system. The muscles are our most pain sensitive organs. Tenderness in the muscle is easily detected on examination. However, alterations in pain perception are not limited to muscles and tendons, they also affect internal organs. That explains why most people with fibromyalgia report bowel pain, bladder pain, and pelvic pain.

The factors involved in the central sensitization of pain in fibromyalgia are being clarified. Compared with people unaffected with the syndrome, patients with fibromyalgia demonstrate exaggerated pain response to direct pressure, to heat, and to electrical stimuli. They are unable to turn off pain signals the way healthy people can, so pain sensations accumulate. This results in an exponential increase in response to pain, termed 'wind up.' At the spinal cord level, nerve receptors that normally are not activated by pain begin to transmit pain, a process called 'allodynia.' Other neurons in the spinal cord become super sensitized. If that isn't enough, there is defective activity of the descending pain modulation system. These mechanisms result in hyperalgesia, an excessive response to a noxious stimulus.

These physiological actions augment the level of pain reaching the brain. There, in the cerebral cortex, past experiences of distress greatly influence the emotional expression of pain. In other areas of the brain the pain response is more fixed, via genetic influences.

Opioid receptors, present in the thalamus, caudate nucleus, and parts of the cerebral cortex, are determined in part by hereditary factors. Specific opioid receptor sites on brain cells in fibromyalgia patients vary from those in healthy control subjects, suggesting that genetic factors are important in the increased pain sensitivity.

Analgesics such as codeine and morphine attach in unique ways to these receptors. Endorphins, our natural opioids, bind to these same receptors. An explosive release of endorphins after acute pain is the presumed mechanism that has allowed American football players run for a touchdown despite a broken ankle. A deficiency of these endogenous opioids alters pain perception. Opioid receptors are present throughout our bodies, in the stomach and the intestine, in muscle and skin, as well as in the brain. Endorphins suppress the body's production of substance P. This pain-generating chemical is important in initiating and maintaining pain. Blocking substance P has been a subject of intense research to help decrease pain. People with fibromyalgia have increased concentrations of substance P in their spinal fluid compared with other people.

Imaging of pain-sensitive areas in the brain, such as the thalamus, have been especially enlightening in understanding central pain mechanisms. Our old friend Sir William Gowers, in 1900, was the first to demonstrate the importance of the thalamus in relaying pain messages. A bullet wound to the thalamus of one of Gowers's patients resulted in total loss of pain sensation. With the advent of functional MRI, positron emission tomography (PET), and single photon emission computed tomography (SPECT) imaging, the neural circuitry of pain is being mapped out. Tiny chemical alterations in response to painful stimuli can be precisely determined. This research has been especially helpful in proving that the pain of fibromyalgia is real. Blood flow to pain-sensitive areas in fibromyalgia patients was lower than that of non-pain control subjects. After painful stimuli, brain blood flow increased more in the patients with fibromyalgia.

Psychological factors affect these dynamic neurological events.

All too often doctors have focused on the emotional factors in chronic pain. The exaggerated pain sensitivity in fibromyalgia has been brushed off as a manifestation of a bruised psyche. Fibromyalgia patients are called hypervigilant. Some of my colleagues still think of people with poorly understood chronic pain, such as in fibromyalgia, as 'wimps.' There may be gender bias here because fibromyalgia is so much more common in 'the weaker sex.' This gender difference may be purely physiological since females of all species have a lower pain threshold than their male counterparts. Cultural expression of pain also varies between the sexes. Men are told to 'be a man.' It is well known that doctors are more likely to attribute pain, for instance from a heart attack, in men to a physiological mechanism while attributing it in women to a psychological mechanism.

We are beginning to understand the environmental influences on pain. Pain response is in part a learned behaviour. Some of us grow up unable to express pain or unwilling to accept it. We are told not to be cry babies. Others grow up embracing pain. The behavioural, cognitive, and socio-cultural variables that influence all forms of pain are being recognized in fibromyalgia. Any two people will respond very differently, i.e., subjectively, to the same pain stimuli. Our response to noxious stimuli is influenced by prior experiences. The autonomic (automatic) nervous system is particularly charged by negative past experiences. For example, one of my patients had been treated with chemotherapy for cancer. Each time she visited her oncologist for a routine checkup she became sick with nausea, fatigue, and severe abdominal cramps. These were the exact symptoms she had experienced during chemotherapy. But now these automatic physical symptoms were triggered by a reawakening of her prior experiences.

The autonomic nervous system is important in pain reactions. Patients with fibromyalgia, as well as those with IBS, demonstrate hyperactivity of the sympathetic portion of the autonomic nervous system. Many of the key nerve cells of the autonomic nervous system are found in the neck, exactly where patients with fibromyalgia have numerous tender points. Blocking nerve fibres of the sympathetic nervous system decreases the pain of fibromyalgia. In contrast, injecting noradrenaline will increase pain sensitivity more in patients with fibromyalgia than in healthy people.

My first goal in working with Jon was to make him understand that his chronic pain was not coming from a structural problem in his spine. It could not be cured by adjustments, injections, or excisions. We talked about the sensitization of pain that happens in the central nervous system. I proposed to decrease pain with medications and to initiate a carefully orchestrated activity and exercise programme. I discontinued the short-acting analgesic that Jon was taking and switched him to a longer acting opioid. The rapid up and down cycles of pain disappeared and he had more lasting pain relief.

Jonathan and I spent the next few months finding ways that would help to remove some of the behaviour maladaptations that he had made to his chronic pain. Bonnie and Jon had purchased three different mattresses during the prior five years, no small financial burden with their marginal income. Hard or soft mattress, three pillows or none, made no difference to Jon's pain. Because he was constantly fearful that he would injure himself, Jon had become increasingly inactive. He was afraid to bend over to tie his shoes. He could not drive for more than ten minutes despite using numerous back supports. Jon had worn a cervical collar and a lumbar corset to no avail. Slowly and grudgingly, Jon began to be more active and more self-reliant. He worked with our physiotherapist twice weekly for the next three months. He began a water exercise programme at the YMCA near his home.

We also talked about his mood and he accepted my suggestion to work with a psychologically trained health professional. The emotional aspects of chronic pain were the most difficult for Jonathan to accept. Jonathan, like anyone with chronic pain, had become conditioned to suffering. Like a wounded animal, he had become cautious, withdrawn, and fearful. He had recognized his depression, but reasoned that this was a normal reaction to chronic pain. I explained that it makes no difference which began first. We know that pain begets depression and depression begets pain. We needed to treat his pain as well as his depression. The addition of an antidepressant lessened his suffering. When I last saw Jon, he was back to part-time work and was taking very few medications. He was coaching his youngest child in softball and was pleased with how far he had come. So was I.

FICTION

- Spinal misalignment is a common cause of back pain and can be mechanically corrected with manipulation.

- An injury or inflammation is the most common cause of chronic pain.

- Pain is real, i.e., physical, or it is purely psychological in origin.

- When the source of pain is not found, people are usually exaggerating their pain.

FACTS

- Back pain is seldom caused by a single structural disorder. Vertebrae and sacroiliac joints do not subluxe. An extensive search for a physical defect in back pain will often be a wild-goose chase.

- Chronic pain takes on a life of its own, not requiring tissue injury or damage; this has been termed 'central sensitization.'

- Our genes, experiences, and environments all contribute to our adaptation to chronic pain. Pain is a physical and emotional sensation.

- Although we can't change inherited biological factors, we can change how we cope with chronic pain.

4

Why Am I Exhausted and Why Can't I Think Straight?

DENISE was forty-five years old when she came to see me in 1995. Her doctor had been puzzled by her profound fatigue, which had been present for four years. A tall, outgoing, attractive brunette, she was immaculately dressed. Her manner and speech were animated. Denise had grown up in Albany, New York. Her father was an insurance agent and her mother an elementary school teacher. One of three children, Denise described her childhood as happy and active. Denise met her husband, Phil, in her final year at college and they were married three years later.

Phil opened a small, successful advertising agency. Shortly after their two children were born, Denise joined Phil's company as an assistant vice-president. The demands on her time occasionally overwhelmed her, but she bounced back quickly with her typical vigour. Then her world came crashing down after a bad bout of the flu in the winter of 1991.

She described her illness to me: *I woke up with a severe sore throat and aches all over. I had a fever for three days and felt so tired that I couldn't get out of bed. My limbs ached terribly. I had no concentration or energy to even watch TV or read a book. My family doctor thought that this was probably flu and prescribed an antibiotic in case I had a throat infection. But I didn't feel any better. After another week of misery, I went back to the doctor for a complete checkup. My glands were swollen, but he couldn't find anything else wrong. All my blood tests were fine.*

Gradually, over the next few months, I felt slightly better, but I couldn't shake the exhaustion. It felt like someone had pulled the plug and that I was totally drained. I tried to keep working, but Phil decided that I should quit. Maybe I had just burned out. I've always demanded a lot of myself and I was always on the go. Now I couldn't accomplish anything. I couldn't fall asleep at night. After a few hours of being up, I needed a nap. The exhaustion began to interfere with my concentration. I could not remember the simplest things.

My body ached everywhere. All of my muscles and skin felt incredibly sensitive when they were touched. If Phil touched me, even tenderly, I couldn't stand it. You can imagine how that made him feel. It started to cause problems between us.

During the next four years I was sent to a number of different specialists, including an infectious disease doctor and a neurologist, but they couldn't find anything suspicious. I kept seeing more and more doctors. I told them that I never got rid of that flu. I was certain that eventually one of these doctors would detect some weird infection and give me a medicine to cure it.

One of the doctors that I saw told me that I was depressed. I agreed to take an antidepressant although I never had been depressed and no one in my family was depressed. My life was fulfilling and happy. The antidepressants made me feel worse. I got jittery and felt confused. I felt helpless. I lost my confidence and my self-esteem, and I was worried that I might lose my husband.

Denise's physical examination was normal, but she was very tender in the typical fibromyalgia locations. I ran various blood tests for anaemia, infections, or thyroid disorders. All of these tests were normal. Like Patty, I felt that Denise had fibromyalgia as well as CFS. I had been working with a CFS expert, Dr. Tony Komaroff, and found that most people with CFS also had fibromyalgia. In many, as with Denise, exhaustion was the overwhelming symptom.

Just like Jon's idiopathic pain, Denise's fatigue had no obvious physical cause. Fatigue is one of the most common complaints that brings people to their doctor. Now and then, everyone has a day or two of fatigue, but 15–20 percent of Americans experience chronic fatigue that persists for months at a time. There are 15 million doctor consultations for fatigue each year in the United States. Fatigue may be caused by medical diseases like thyroid deficiency, anaemia, arthritis, or immune disorders. Depression is another common reason for people to be exhausted. But often no apparent disease is found. Blood tests and physical examinations are unrevealing. This idiopathic chronic fatigue has been given various names during the past century, most recently chronic fatigue syndrome.

Diagnostic criteria for what we now call chronic fatigue syndrome have been established and, as in fibromyalgia, these criteria are based on symptoms. The cardinal symptom of CFS is chronic, debilitating fatigue that persists or relapses for more than six months. Other medical and psychiatric disorders that cause chronic fatigue must be excluded. Patients diagnosed with CFS must also have four or more of the following: muscle pain, multijoint pain, impaired memory or concentration, new headaches, unrefreshing sleep, post-exertion malaise, sore throat, and tender lymph nodes in the neck or arm. Generally the physical examination and blood tests are normal. Laboratory testing does not contribute to CFS diagnosis except to exclude other conditions.

The rather arbitrary nature of defining syndromes is exemplified with CFS. It is important that CFS can be distinguished from depression, and it was also hoped that CFS diagnostic criteria would focus on its potential infectious etiology. The initial CFS criteria were too restrictive. You could not have depression and also be classified as having CFS, which made no sense. Depression is present in many chronic diseases. The 'infectious' symptoms of the CFS definition are fever, swollen glands, and sore throat. These are only 'minor' criteria and you can be diagnosed with CFS without manifesting any of these markers of infection.

When epidemiologists used the more restrictive CFS definition, they estimated that there were about 400,000 cases of CFS in the United States. A more liberal case definition of CFS found ten times that number. Physicians throughout the world recognize that unexplained chronic fatigue is one of the most common symptoms in medicine. The controversy is whether a subset of CFS sufferers has a different, definable disorder. Any case definition is operational, meaning it is being tested and subject to change. Operational criteria provide the foundation for investigators to study a group of symptoms in the population.

I told Denise that she had CFS. She also had fibromyalgia. Around 70 percent of CFS patients also meet the diagnostic criteria for fibromyalgia. A Canadian report found that 60 percent of fibromyalgia patients met criteria for CFS. CFS and fibromyalgia may be the same illness or their symptoms may co-exist. If a patient has both fibromyalgia and CFS, they tend to have worse health and a poorer outcome than people who only have CFS.

Like fibromyalgia, CFS is not new. Doctors keep changing their positions on CFS just as in fibromyalgia. What we now call chronic fatigue syndrome was described in 1750 by Sir Richard Manningham. His patients reported, 'profound listlessness, with great lassitude and weariness all over the body and little, flying pains.' The American neurologist Dr. George Beard chose the name 'neurasthenia' in 1869 since he believed that the illness was caused by a 'weakness of the nerves and nervous exhaustion.' Beard described a similar dilemma that I faced with Denise while attempting to decipher the complexities of her exhaustion: 'The diagnosis of neurasthenia is obtained partly by the positive symptoms and partly by exclusion. It may be associated with almost every conceivable form of organic disease. In such cases it is sometimes very difficult to ascertain whether it is the cause or the effect. The history of the symptoms will help us to decide this question.' Beard also recognized that pressures of modern civilization increased the exhaustion, writing, 'A person with a nervous tendency is driven to think, to work, to strive for success. He presses himself and his life forces to the limit, straining his circuits. Like an overloaded battery . . . the sufferer's electrical system crashes down, spewing sparks and symptoms and giving rise to neurasthenia.'

During most of the past century, doctors have debated whether CFS is an infectious disease. Clusters of cases of what we now call CFS were described in the 1930s, 1940s, and 1950s throughout the world. In 1934, an outbreak of an illness identical to the current descriptions of CFS occurred in health-care workers at Los Angeles County General Hospital. The polio virus was then rampant, and public health experts suspected that an atypical form of polio was the culprit. Newspapers in Los Angeles played up the public health threat of this 'new epidemic,' comparing it with polio. However, the neurological symptoms were milder, no paralysis ever developed, and no virus was detected. The single, most common chronic symptom in these patients was exhaustion, often lasting for years. Over the next fifty years, cases of chronic, unexplained fatigue occurred in several clusters of people throughout the world. Large outbreaks were reported in Iceland, South Africa, England, and Australia. The 'epidemic' nature of these cases again suggested that an infectious agent was involved. However, no infection turned up in the vast majority of the patients, and no patients died or became paralyzed.

Then, in 1984, an epidemic of unexplained fatigue, called a 'mysterious, new disease,' was reported among residents of Incline Village, Nevada. Most people also had a variety of symptoms that included muscle aches, headaches, diarrhoea, dizziness, numbness, tingling, and weakness. Two studies published in prestigious medical journals suggested that the virus that causes infectious mononucleosis ('mono'), the Epstein-Barr virus (EBV), might be the culprit. Incriminating the Epstein-Barr virus was logical.

Infectious mononucleosis causes exhaustion that may persist for months. The EBV, like other herpes viruses, remains dormant in our blood long after apparent infections. Most important, studies in Nevada reported elevated Epstein-Barr virus antibody levels in the blood of these chronically fatigued patients, suggesting a recent infection.

However, the specificity of these elevated antibody levels to the Epstein-Barr virus was questioned by more investigations. A team of epidemiologists from the U.S. Centers for Disease Control (CDC) found no evidence that this new illness was a specific disease. Further research at medical centres throughout the world during the next ten years found no link between CFS and viral infection. Early hopes that a cause for chronic fatigue would be found gradually faded in both patients and investigators, but particularly the latter. The notion that CFS was a 'disease' was again questioned. Some physicians argued that CFS was nothing more than anxiety and hysteria.

Denise was certain that her chronic fatigue had been caused by flu four years before. I told her that an infection could have triggered her symptoms, but it was highly unlikely that after all this time, an infectious agent was actively involved. I told her that antibiotics or antiviral drugs were unlikely to improve her symptoms. Denise turned to a CFS support group for help. She was given the name of a CFS expert who was 'curing the infection that caused CFS.' Denise explained, *I had to find a doctor who could find the cause of my CFS. I was sure that I had some strange infection. Would I infect my husband and children? Living with me became a nightmare for my family. I was afraid to kiss my husband or kids. Every time anyone had a cough or a cold, I isolated myself from the rest of my family. The doctor recommended by the support group founded a CFS clinic. He prescribed antibiotics to kill a bacteria called mycoplasma (bacteria that he said caused my illness). But after one month of this treatment, I felt just as miserable. Then I got intravenous kutapressin and interferon to boost my immune system. I felt less tired for a week, but came home no better.*

I next went to a holistic physician who ran an 'allergy-immunology clinic.' This doctor told me that my blood, urine, and skin tests proved that I was infected with both the Epstein-Barr virus and yeast. Based on these tests, I was diagnosed with Chronic Fatigue Immune Dysfunction Syndrome. His clinic put me on a strict 'elimination diet.' Desensitizing injections were used to rid my body of various toxins. I also was given antifungal and antibacterial medicines.

My blood tests and skin tests also demonstrated allergies to a large number of pollens, foods, and chemicals. The clinic staff thought that my symptoms may have begun when I was working in a new building a few years earlier. A number of other workers on my floor had become ill and there was concern that the ventilation system in the building was leaking harmful fumes. At that point they told me that I also had the multiple chemical sensitivity syndrome.

My lifestyle became very confined since I was convinced that germs and chemicals would make me worse. I was worried about going out of the house. All of the tests and most of the treatments were not covered by my medical insurance and I spent thousands of dollars. The elimination diet greatly restricted what I could eat and I lost twenty pounds that I couldn't afford to lose. When their treatment was done, I weighed only a hundred pounds and looked like I had stepped out of a concentration camp. But I was still totally exhausted. My memory got so bad that I thought that I was getting Alzheimer's disease. One day I went to the cupboard to get a cup for my daughter, and I couldn't remember the word 'cup.'

Like Denise, most people with fibromyalgia and CFS report mental confusion and memory loss. These cognitive disturbances have been referred to as 'fibro fog.' People often stumble for words. Mental tasks that require rapid thoughts, such as simple maths, are especially difficult. Denise was very worried that she was becoming demented. Her aunt had developed Alzheimer's disease at the age of fifty-five. The cognitive disturbances reported in fibromyalgia and CFS are not progressive and not related to dementia. They are quite similar to the cognitive problems that develop after head injuries. Susan, a patient referred to me last year for fibromyalgia, described memory problems similar to those of Denise.

Susan was healthy until she was involved in a motor-vehicle accident six years earlier. She reported, *I was stopped at a red light and a car slammed into the back of my car. My head snapped forwards and then I developed severe pain in my head and neck. X-rays were normal and I was treated with muscle relaxants, but the pain really never went away. Over the next few years, the pain spread to my shoulders and arms and my chest. All the time, I had difficulty concentrating. I couldn't remember simple things or process complicated information. Frequently I would feel dizzy, especially when I would get up in the morning. Sometimes the room was spinning. When I was walking I often lost my equilibrium. Gradually the slightest noise would start increasing my dizziness and headaches. My neck became so tight that I couldn't turn around when I was backing up in the drive.*

A few months ago I was driving home and all of a sudden I got lost. I recognized the neighbourhood, but I couldn't figure out where I was or how I got there. I called my husband frantically. Then we both got really worried and I had a complete neurological examination. My MRI was okay. I spent two days undergoing psychiatric and neuropsychological examinations. They told me that the tests were consistent with 'post-concussion brain damage.'

Dr. Simon Wessely described the cognitive disturbances in CFS as '. . . the patient needs to devote more attention or even energy to motor and cognitive tasks, such as muscular exertion or mental concentration. Previously automatic tasks require higher levels of vigilance and thus become effortful.' The fatigue present in people with fibromyalgia and CFS is multidimensional, represented by physical, psychological, cognitive, and behavioural disturbances.

Susan was prescribed methylphenidate (Ritalin) for the attention problems and sertraline (Lustral) to treat her fatigue. Gradually, she noted better concentration and less irritability, although her short-term memory is still not as good as she thinks it should be.

CFS and fibromyalgia are associated with cognitive disturbances, muscle pain, and exhaustion. In much of the world, including the United Kingdom, CFS has been called benign myalgic encephalomyelitis, 'myalgic' to account for the muscle pain and 'encephalomyelitis' to account for involvement of the brain. Indeed, CFS and fibromyalgia are now viewed as illnesses of the nervous system. This does not mean that irreversible brain damage occurs. The most terrifying myth regarding CFS is that it inexorably destroys brain tissue. Hillary Johnson wrote in her book *Osler's Web,* 'CFS is an infectious disease that can devastate the immune system, attack the brain, and leave its victims physically and emotionally overwhelmed.' Such statements are scientifically misleading. No immune deficiency or brain disease occurs. Nevertheless, physiological (dynamic) abnormalities, similar to fibromyalgia, are present in CFS.

MRIs of the brain demonstrate small 'signal abnormalities' in the white matter in some CFS patients. In some respects, such changes are similar to the plaques found on an MRI study of patients with multiple sclerosis. But, in contrast to multiple sclerosis, there is no evidence that such brain changes are permanent or progressive. Furthermore, such abnormalities on MRI and related changes on SPECT scans are also seen in patients with fibromyalgia, migraine, and even in 20–30 percent of healthy people. Nevertheless, Denise had been told that irreversible brain damage occurs and the MRI and SPECT scan abnormalities proved it.

Dynamic blood flow changes are present in fibromyalgia and CFS. Dynamic means fluctuating and reversible. It does not imply permanent or progressive. These dynamic fluctuations are influenced by neurohormones such as serotonin, corticotrophin-releasing hormone (CRH), and noradrenaline. A deficiency of these hormones results in debilitating fatigue, muscle and joint pain, and disturbances in sleep and mood. Therefore, I tried Denise on a low dose of sertraline (Lustral) to see if her energy might pick up. The SSRI antidepressants like fluoxetine (Prozac) or sertraline (Lustral) may help to decrease the fatigue by enhancing serotonin levels.

There is no evidence that CFS is associated with major immune deficiency. In contrast to immune deficiency states such as HIV infection or certain forms of cancer, people with CFS never develop life-threatening opportunistic infections. They do not demonstrate the very low levels of T-cell lymphocytes that characterize immune dysfunction. Based on the false assumption that CFS is a viral-induced immune disease, megavitamins, immune enhancers, and antiviral agents have each been used for treatment. Not surprisingly, they have not been beneficial.

Nevertheless, subtle immune alterations have been found in a subset of CFS and fibromyalgia patients. Decreased numbers of specific T-cell lymphocytes that kill viruses, as well as activation of certain enzymes that are triggered during viral infection, suggests a chronic low-level immune war. The significance of such immune system findings is unclear.

Denise was thin and her blood pressure was low. She often felt faint when she got out of bed or out of a chair quickly. I checked her blood pressure and pulse when she was lying down, sitting, and standing. Her blood pressure dropped and her heart rate increased more than expected. This is called orthostatic intolerance. Denise, as had many of my patients, reported other symptoms often associated with postural hypotension. These included light-headedness, 'fuzziness,' dizziness, difficulty focusing and concentrating, cold hands and feet, and mottling of her skin. Fainting or near-fainting with rapid changes in posture is the cardinal symptom of orthostatic intolerance, but these other symptoms can be part of the picture.

Patients with CFS and fibromyalgia are prone to fainting with rapid changes in body position. Such fainting represents an exaggerated response of the autonomic nervous system. An abnormal heart rate response to body position, or other stressors, in a patient with fibromyalgia, indicates that there is excess sympathetic nervous system activity. Denise underwent tilt table testing, which confirmed that she was excessively intolerant to abrupt changes in posture. Recognition of orthostatic (postural) intolerance in fibromyalgia and CFS has promoted more research on the autonomic nervous system. The exact relationship of fatigue with low blood pressure is unclear. Initially we were enthusiastic about treating CFS and fibromyalgia patients who had orthostatic intolerance with drugs, such as fluorinated steroids that raise the blood pressure response. I tried this to no avail with Denise and recent clinical trials with this approach were equally disappointing. Denise is now careful to drink a lot of water, use salt, and avoid dehydration.

As with fibromyalgia, the medical profession is divided regarding the nature of CFS. Many believe that fibromyalgia and CFS are primarily cultural phenomena. Their acceptance by society varies with the times. Excess 'female sickliness' has been correlated with thwarted ambitions of women in society. Some social scientists contend that the medical and cultural acceptability of CFS has paralleled times of major role changes for women. They conclude that CFS is more likely to occur in the 'weaker sex' because of excess pressure on women. Even feminist authors have linked neurasthenia and CFS to women's distress and lack of satisfaction in life. For the nineteenth-century physician, this was felt to cause 'depletion of our limited supply of nervous energy' (a literal translation of 'neurasthenia').

Doctors can argue over the name or the cause of CFS and fibromyalgia. What they must not argue over is the distress that these illnesses cause. There is a tendency to presume that disability and suffering are less real when no observable disease is present. Doctors, patients, and the media need to stop searching for absolutes and concentrate on the many facets of chronic illness. The old biochemical model of disease does not work well with fibromyalgia and CFS. One of my colleagues, Dr. Komaroff, wrote: 'CFS may become a paradigmatic illness that leads us away from being trapped by the rigidity of the conventional biomedical model and lead us to a fuller understanding of suffering.'

During the past year, Denise's energy improved and she became much more active. She gradually accepted the notion that we could help her suffering even if we did not know its cause or cure. Last year she said: *Once I accepted that I could get better without knowing why I got sick, I felt relieved. It was important to get on with my life and forget about searching for the infection that must be inside me. My husband began to come to our discussion and treatment sessions, which was very important to me. I felt that he had not been too supportive of my situation. He admitted that after all the years of me being ill while looking healthy and doctors not finding anything, he had begun to question the reality of my illness. During the past year, our relationship improved greatly. We began to do much more together and were much happier. I've got my life back.*

FICTION

■ **CFS and fibromyalgia are not specific illnesses, but 'dustbin terms' given to people who are not coping well with life.**

■ **CFS and fibromyalgia are different diseases.**

■ **CFS is caused by an infection and results in immune deficiency.**

■ **CFS and fibromyalgia cause progressive damage to the brain.**

■ **CFS should be treated with antimicrobial drugs and therapy to bolster a failing immune system.**

FACTS

- CFS is defined by its symptoms, primarily debilitating fatigue in the absence of another disease.

- The majority of people who have CFS also have fibromyalgia.

- There is no evidence that an infection or immune deficit causes CFS or fibromyalgia.

- Fatigue and cognitive disturbances are related to a number of physiological changes in the central nervous system and the autonomic nervous system. These are reversible. Dementia or progressive damage does not occur.

- The treatments of CFS and fibromyalgia are similar.

5

Why Do I Have Constant Headaches?

SCOTT, a thirty-nine-year-old computer engineer, had suffered from migraine headaches since he was fourteen. However, during the past few years he began having different and constant headaches that triggered pain in his neck, shoulders, and back. In the six months before I examined Scott, he noted constant, dull pain throughout his upper body, but most pronounced in his head and neck. His family doctor thought that the headaches were due to arthritis of his neck and referred Scott to me.

Scott told me that his headaches were often brought on by stress. He said, *I have always been intense and very goal directed. My father was a scientist and my mother owned a jewellery store. When I was young, I was a self-sufficient, only child. My grades were excellent and I went to university when I was seventeen. Other than belonging to a university society and the usual weekend parties, I wasn't much for social events. But in my last year of college, I met Jennifer and we got married the next year.*

We have three children and our lives are busy with their schedules and our work. I'm now one of the senior people in our company. I'm travelling too much, including overseas trips, each month. I often feel burned out and my headaches get much worse when I overwork. But I don't know how to relax! Every time I plan to start an exercise programme, something comes up. Jennifer has been trying to get me to stop working so hard, but I enjoy my job. Troubleshooting all over the country is invigorating. But lately I have been travelling three days in every week. I'm usually up by 5 a.m., in the office by 6.30 when I'm not out of town. I make it a point to be home for dinner with the kids, but I usually work at home until late.

Scott was short, overweight, and serious in nature. He was quite introspective and had obviously given a lot of thought to his illness. We immediately got along well, especially because he shared my passion for films. I also identified closely with Scott because of my own experiences with incapacitating headaches.

Scott described the migraines that he began experiencing as a teenager. *From the ages of fourteen to nineteen, I got a headache at least once each month. First I would see zig-zag lines and flashing lights. That was my signal that the headache was ready to explode. Then my forehead and temple started to pound – like my pulse. If I didn't take pain medication quickly and lie down, the headache became terrible and I would miss a few days of school. I could never figure out what brought on the headaches, except sometimes bright lights would start them. All of a sudden during my second year in college, the migraines went away. I was headache-free for years.*

Three years ago, just a few weeks after I had root canal surgery, I began getting headaches again. But they were different, constant and boring across my forehead. The headaches were accompanied by pain and spasm in my neck. A burning sensation radiated down my right arm. My whole neck and arm became so tight that I could barely turn my head enough to drive my car.

Thinking that his headaches were probably related to the root canal surgery, Scott went back to his dentist, who diagnosed temporomandibular joint syndrome (TMJ). Scott was referred to a dental school maxillo-facial clinic that specialized in TMJ. His subsequent dental examination revealed clicking and some malalignment of the right jaw. Some of the specialists told Scott that jaw surgery would alleviate the headache, but others disagreed. Scott was treated with anti-inflammatory medicines, gentle jaw exercises, and physical therapy. At night he wore a mouth guard to prevent him from grinding his teeth. But Scott's jaw pain and headaches persisted. After another year of misery, Scott decided to have the jaw reconstructive surgery.

But Scott, like Jon, found that surgery was not the answer. He told me, *Since the jaw operation, the headaches are worse. I can't concentrate enough to work. It feels like my head is in a vice. I can't move my head or neck from side to side. When the headaches aren't controlled with pain medicine, it feels like my forehead is going to explode. The pain travels in a band across my head and temples and down my neck. Both of my shoulders and arms are very tender. Lately my upper and middle back have been killing me.*

A chiropractor told Scott that the headaches were related to a subluxation of the vertebrae in his neck. Chiropractic spinal manipulation during the next three months only made Scott's headaches worse. He then went to see a neurologist. An MRI of his neck and head revealed some disc space narrowing, but there was no spinal cord compression. The neurologist told Scott that he did not feel that these findings explained his headaches or his neck pain. He could not give Scott a diagnosis but told him 'it is muscular.' He prescribed cervical traction, which helped Scott's neck pain slightly, but did not help the headaches.

When I examined Scott he was exquisitely tender in the muscles on the right side of his face and neck and throughout his upper back. Deep pressure in some of his neck muscles caused pain to radiate down Scott's arm. This referred pain sensation is characteristic of a 'trigger point.' He also had tender points in his upper back and shoulder muscles. The rest of his examination was unremarkable. I reviewed Scott's neck and back X-rays as well as brain and spine MRIs, all of which were normal.

I told Scott that his headaches, muscle pain, and tenderness fitted the picture of a localized form of fibromyalgia, termed 'myofascial pain syndrome.' The headaches were related to chronic muscle contractions in his head and neck, so-called tension headaches. I explained that 50 percent of patients with fibromyalgia and myofascial pain also suffer from migraine headaches and more than 70 percent from muscular headaches. In Scott's case, headaches were his major problem. Nevertheless, he had all of the other symptoms of fibromyalgia.

Here, too, terminology has been controversial. Myofascial pain syndrome implies that the muscle pain and tender points are localized to one region of the body, often the head and neck. In contrast, fibromyalgia is defined by widespread muscle pain. Sometimes, such as following a motor-vehicle accident or other trauma, pain seems to begin locally and then spreads. It is not uncommon for a person to have myofascial pain initially, but eventually full-blown fibromyalgia. TMJ is another name for myofascial pain of the jaw and face region. Of fibromyalgia patients, 94 percent report TMJ.

Some oral surgeons and dentists claim that TMJ is usually caused by a malalignment of the jaw. They advise wearing a mouthguard at night to prevent grinding of the teeth. If that doesn't work, surgical intervention to correct the jaw malalignment is performed. Too often such surgery is not the answer because there is no correctable bone or joint damage. Surgery did not cure Scott's head and neck pain.

Many doctors believe that fibromyalgia and myofascial pain are separable. They distinguish the trigger points of myofascial pain from the tender points of fibromyalgia. They point to studies demonstrating changes in muscle electrical discharge at these trigger points.

Many of the concepts about myofascial pain syndrome follow the teaching of Dr. Janet Travell. Dr. Travell, a brilliant specialist in physical medicine, was John F. Kennedy's personal doctor and the first female White House physician. She popularized the notion that trigger points refer pain to other parts of the body in reproducible patterns. She advised vigorous local treatment such as spraying the muscle with a topical anaesthetic and stretching it. Travell and her advocates suggest that myofascial pain and fibromyalgia have different origins and require different therapy.

However, investigations that I did with Drs. Fred Wolfe, Rob Bennett, Travell, and a number of myofascial pain experts found no significant differences in the symptoms and physical findings of patients with fibromyalgia and myofascial pain. Both cause muscle tenderness and both syndromes refer pain down the belly of the muscle. Often this referred pain is associated with numbness, tingling, or burning sensations.

Most of my colleagues and I believe that myofascial pain is best considered to be a more localized form of fibromyalgia. I diagnose myofascial pain when the muscle pain is limited to one region of the body such as the head and neck. However, often this more focal myofascial pain will gradually spread to become the widespread pain of fibromyalgia. Early recognition and treatment may halt its spread to a more generalized fibromyalgia. However, sometimes myofascial pain extends into fibromyalgia despite the best treatment. The basic mechanisms of abnormal pain perception discussed in fibromyalgia and chronic back pain apply to myofascial pain.

During the next year Scott's muscular headaches slowly improved. Physical exercises and stretching eased the neck pain. Scott also was taught relaxation techniques such as meditation. He was headache-free for more than a year. We talked on the phone twice, primarily about new film recommendations. Unfortunately, Scott returned to see me last year a few days after having, as he called it, 'the worst migraine of my life.' His description of the migraine conjured up dreadful recollections of my own headaches. He described these explicitly: *It began with a dull ache over my right temple and forehead. When I was younger my migraines were always preceded by visual signs – the aura. This one wasn't, but I felt the same overwhelming sense of dread.*

Within an hour the head pain was severe and I felt sick. The headache was pounding and my scalp was tender when I touched it. The pain decreased when I compressed the artery that was pounding at my temple. I could not stand any light or sound. I had to lie down in a dark room with no noise. First I felt warm and flushed. Then I got cold and clammy. As the headache subsided, a sense of dread and anxiety washed over me. For the next twelve hours I was irritable and depressed. Finally, the migraine went away only to be followed by another one a few days later.

I knew first-hand what Scott was describing. During the past ten years I would get a migraine headache like Scott's every few months. Then I would spend days trying to figure out why the headache had come on. Scott and I both searched high and low for a structural cause for our headaches. There was none to be found.

Two out of three Americans report at least one bothersome headache each month. Each year in the United States there are 18 million medical visits for evaluation and treatment of headaches. Headaches are the most common symptom that brings people to see a physician. At some time, 50 percent of women and 40 percent of men will experience a headache severe enough that they cannot work. As with fibromyalgia and CFS, the exact cause of most headaches is not known. Very occasionally, headaches may be an early sign of a serious underlying illness such as cancer, stroke, or infection. These diseases usually can be quickly diagnosed, especially with advances in diagnostic imaging such as the MRI. However, the vast majority of headaches are not caused by a systemic disease or brain damage.

Headaches, like fibromyalgia, are diagnosed based on a patient's symptoms. Once again, the physical examination, X-rays, and blood tests are used only to exclude structural disease. There is no diagnostic gold standard. The two most common headaches are classified as muscular or 'tension' headaches and vascular or migraine headaches. There is marked overlap between such headaches. For lack of a better term, most people with muscle-type headaches are told they have 'tension headaches.' This implies that their pain is a manifestation of 'psychic tension.' No solid research supports this theory. There is no evidence that people with muscular headaches have more psychological stress or more psychiatric illness than people without headaches. Among fibromyalgia patients, 70–90 percent report frequent muscular headaches.

Migraine comes from the term 'hemi-cranium' or 'half skull' since it is usually most intense over one temple. Migraine headaches are described as 'vascular' because of their throbbing, pulse-like quality. They are subdivided into classic migraine, with visual hallucinations or aura, and common migraine, without aura. Scott's headaches when he was young were classic migraine, and the recent ones were the common migraine type. In the United States, 20 million women and 10 million men get migraine. Nearly half of these migraine sufferers experience moderate to severe disability. The cost from lost work productivity due to headaches in the United States is as high as $17 billion per year.

Migraine was first described in 3000 B.C. and has afflicted many famous and infamous figures, including Julius Caesar and Sigmund Freud. Hippocrates in 400 B.C. described migraine headaches in one of his patients: 'Most of the time he seemed to see something shining before him like a light, usually in part of the right eye. At the end of a moment, a violent pain supervened in the right temple, then in all the head and neck, where the head is attached to the spine.' However, for centuries migraine was considered to be a psychogenic illness. Theories abounded that neuroses, maybe associated with hormonal changes in women, were largely responsible for migraine. Freud's profound impact on neurology and psychiatry promoted the notion that migraine was a psychic phenomenon.

Like fibromyalgia and CFS, migraine is a systemic illness with symptoms involving every organ of the body. These symptoms run the gamut from nausea, vomiting, diarrhoea, abdominal pain, dizziness, exhaustion, and mood disturbances. A migraine attack may mimic a stroke with the onset of temporary blindness or loss of speech. Some of the more bizarre symptoms include vertigo, eyelid drooping, watery eyes, runny nose, facial swelling, or nose-bleeds. Migraine, like fibromyalgia, is a bio-psychological illness. Neurologist Oliver Sacks, who wrote *The Man Who Mistook His Wife for a Hat* and *Awakenings* (made into a film), described the interplay of the mind and body. 'A migraine is a physical event that may also from the start or later become an emotional or symbolic event. A migraine expresses both physiological and emotional needs: it is the prototype of a psychophysiological reaction.'

At the onset of a migraine, physical symptoms usually dominate. The headaches are associated with sensitivity to light, photophobia, and to noise, phonophobia. The migraine aura, a phantasm of visual hallucinations, represents a microcosm of neurological symptoms. The aura often consists of zig-zag lines with flashes of brilliant light and geometric shapes. These may obscure vision. Often with migraines, paraesthesias (as in fibromyalgia) that feel like a burning or a loss of sensation will spread over a limb to the face. Clumsiness or even temporary paralysis of a limb may follow the attack. Emotional symptoms including depression, apathy, and social withdrawal then take over.

Often, the mood changes accompanying migraine are profound. Overwhelming fatigue, a sense of terror, and a sudden and deep depression follow or sometimes precede the headache. Scott felt emotionally drained for hours after his migraine. The depression associated with migraine usually occurs suddenly, without external emotional stress, and resolves within minutes or hours. I know of no other illness that so suddenly transforms a perfectly healthy and happy person to a physical and emotional wreck.

Scott experienced a migraine headache at least once a week during the next three months. He was unable to continue working. He also became depressed. I identified closely with Scott since I, too, became depressed after my headaches had persisted for months.

The association of depression and migraine works in two ways. As in fibromyalgia, the pain and uncertainty of migraine headaches cause a reactive depression. Pain causes worry and pessimism, and impairs function. Migraine and depression also share certain causal factors. If you have a past history of depression, you are at greater risk of getting attacks of migraine. This is also true for fibromyalgia. Biological and genetic factors predispose a person to migraine, fibromyalgia, and depression. In some families with many members affected with migraine, the genetic pattern of inheritance has been mapped out. Fibromyalgia and migraine both occur more frequently in women. They are both affected by changes in oestrogen. Before puberty there are similar rates of migraine in boys and girls, but after puberty migraine is three times as common in females. Some women have an attack of migraine only at the onset of their menstrual cycle, whereas others may get an attack when they ovulate. Stress, too much or too little exercise, certain foods, lack of sleep, dehydration, bright lights, or strong odours may precipitate an attack of migraine. Note the clinical similarities to fibromyalgia.

There is decreased blood flow to certain parts of the brain at the onset of a migraine headache. Such dynamic shifts in cerebral blood flow are similar to what I have described in fibromyalgia and CFS. A diminished blood supply to the brain hemisphere is observed at regions where the headaches are most intense. The reduced blood supply is associated with changes in electrical discharges of brain cells, referred to as the spreading cortical depression of Leao. There is also increased blood flow in the brain stem, an area rich in serotonin. Patients with severe migraine demonstrate higher serotonin synthesis in many regions of their brains. The release of serotonin at the site of a migraine causes constriction of cerebral arteries, impeding the normal blood flow. Levels of serotonin and the metabolites of serotonin in platelets, plasma, urine, and cerebrospinal fluid are different in patients with migraine compared with normal individuals. Serotonin alterations are important in migraine, depression, and in fibromyalgia.

Many of the pharmacological agents used to treat migraine interact with serotonin. Some of the most specific and most effective medications yet developed for migraine include the triptans, such as sumatriptan (Imigran), which is a serotonin receptor ago-nist or activator. Methysergide, which also works at the site of serotonin receptors, is often used for the prophylaxis of attacks of migraine. The tricyclic antidepressants, such as amitriptyline, and the SSRIs, such as fluoxetine (Prozac) and sertraline (Lustral), may also be useful in the treatment of migraine. Nitrous oxide, laugh-ing gas, has been used as an analgesic and an anaesthetic for the past century. One of its effects is to increase cerebral blood flow. It has recently been found to be of some efficacy in the treatment of acute migraine. Research in fibromyalgia has demonstrated enhanced brain synthesis of nitrous oxide.

Drug therapy is more targeted and more effective in migraine than for muscular headaches or fibromyalgia. Muscular headaches are usually treated with pain relievers (analgesics), NSAIDs, or antidepressant medications as used in the treatment of fibromyal-gia. Medications to treat migraine come in two types: those that prevent attacks and those that abort an attack that has already begun. Preventing attacks of migraine should be considered if the attacks are frequent and debilitating. Examples of preventive migraine medicines include the beta blockers, such as propanolol; calcium channel blockers, such as verapamil; and the old standby, tricyclic antidepressants, such as amitriptyline.

Sumatriptan (Imigran) and the newer triptans abort an attack of migraine before it becomes full-blown. They block the neurohormonal-mediated pain response and relax constricted blood vessels. Other medications that can reduce the severity of migraine include NSAIDs, steroids, various narcotic analgesics, and ergot derivatives. Ergot is a fungus that infects rye plants. Its effects on the human nervous system can be helpful or harmful, depending on how it is administered. In migraine, dihydroergota-mine is most popular, given by self-administered injections. Scott's migraine responded very well to Imigran (sumatriptan). He had only three more attacks over the next six months and each sub-sided within an hour or two of taking the drug.

A better scientific understanding of the action of drugs for treating migraine has helped put to rest the age-old debate about the mind or the body in migraine. As in fibromyalgia and CFS, the increased prevalence of migraine in women may have heightened the fantasy that migraine was purely a psychogenic illness. Oliver Sacks described the historical illusion of a migraineur as 'ambitious, successful, perfectionistic, rigid, cautious, and emotionally constipated, driven therefore from time to time to outbursts and breakdowns that must assume an indirect, somatic form.'

Most doctors have changed their views and now acknowledge that migraine is a neuro-biological, not a psychogenic, disorder. Neurologists have led the way. Ironically, neurologists have been the most vocal critics of fibromyalgia. Neurologists continue to embrace the idea that migraine is a physical illness, but consider fibromyalgia to be a psychological disorder. The similar clinical and physiological findings suggest that is not so.

Scott used stress reduction methods to treat his fibromyalgia headaches. He enrolled in our ten week stress reduction programme for patients with fibromyalgia (See Table on Treatment, page 134). This programme includes elements of cognitive behavioural therapy as well as meditation and yoga. The aim of cognitive behavioural therapy is to alter negative thoughts and to foster healthier ways to adapt to illness. We use a combination of theory teaching sessions followed by rehearsal and maintenance programmes to achieve these goals.

The cognitive behavioural portion focuses on our patients' daily activities and their time commitments, and provides ways for them to stop and think rather than to constantly be doing. Feelings of helplessness and hopelessness are rooted out. Meditation and simple yoga is taught in group sessions and practised daily by each patient. The efficacy of such a programme compares favourably with the results of our fibromyalgia medication studies with drugs such as amitriptyline and fluoxetine (Prozac).

I asked Scott to modify his work schedule. He had long recognized the toll that his workload had on him, but he had never been able to let go of much responsibility. Scott could not delegate work to others. Except for his love of films, he had very few hobbies or interests. Family holidays always included his laptop computer and mobile phone. Scott would constantly be in touch with his office, whether in Japan or at a family social occasion.

He described how he learned to control his headaches: *As soon as I have an inkling of a migraine, I stop what I am doing and go to a quiet room. I turn off the lights and shut my eyes and begin to focus on my breathing. Breathing slowly and deeply, I feel my stomach and chest expand, then relax. Each out breath encourages a sense of letting go. I think about relaxing every part of my body, starting with my toes and moving up to my head. By the time I reach my head, the tension in my forehead and around my eyes has noticeably lessened. If I still feel my pulse around my temples pounding, I imagine that the pulse is becoming softer and quieter. Finally, I will picture a calm scene such as a clear mountain lake. Sometimes my relaxation techniques work so well that I don't take the migraine medicine. The breathing and imagery have become a good way for me to relax at any time, even if I'm not getting a headache. They have become a 'preventive medicine' for me.*

Doctors often view headaches, like fibromyalgia, as a nuisance. Many doctors consider that the evaluation and treatment of headaches occupy more of our time than is warranted. Diagnosis is elusive. Treatment is inadequate. As with fibromyalgia and back pain, patients are told that they 'must learn to live with it.' Because headaches are so prevalent and so often discounted by doctors, people often turn to alternative or non-traditional treatments such as herbs and nutritional supplements. But as the physiological underpinnings of headaches are better understood, treatment is becoming much more effective.

FICTION

- Migraine is a vascular headache that is biologically distinct from muscle headaches and conditions like fibromyalgia.

- Myofascial pain is caused by chemical or structural muscle changes, in contrast to fibromyalgia.

- TMJ is a structural jaw disorder.

- Objective evidence for an organic disease is present in migraine, but not in tension headaches or in fibromyalgia.

FACTS

- Physiological changes in migraine are similar to those in fibromyalgia. Of fibromyalgia patients, 70 percent suffer from chronic muscular headaches and 50 percent from migraine.

- Muscle headaches and facial and jaw pain are characteristic of myofascial pain syndrome, a localized form of fibromyalgia.

- Structural problems of the head and neck rarely cause chronic pain and headaches.

- Genetic, psychological, gender, and biological factors are important in migraine and are similar to those in fibromyalgia. Treatment principles are similar.

6

What About My Bowel and Bladder Irritability?

JANE, a twenty-one-year-old student, began having attacks of muscle and joint pain during her last year of school. She also had a life-long history of abdominal cramping with alternating constipation and diarrhoea. Jane told me: *I have had stomach problems since I was five. I have always been either constipated or get diarrhoea, often with severe cramps. Sometimes the pains were so bad I had to stay home from school. My mother had ulcerative colitis and I was told at nine that I probably had that, too. However, over the next few years I had several examinations, including a biopsy of my intestine. The doctors then said that I did not have ulcerative colitis, but they didn't know what was wrong.*

When I was twelve, a holistic-type doctor told me that I had chronic parasite infections. My stools were sent to a special laboratory in Montana. The doctor recommended a wheat-free and sugar-free diet and treatment with antibiotics. My gut felt no better. Eventually, I think to get rid of me, a gastroenterologist told me that I had irritable bowel syndrome. He said I needed to relax more and not take life so seriously. At that point, doctors stopped taking much interest in me.

Jane was an outstanding student and athlete at school. A superb gymnast, at the age of eleven Jane had considered moving to Texas to train for the Olympics. While at school, she had few friends and rarely dated. She did very well academically and was accepted at a U.S. Ivy League college. However, in her first year of college, she lost fifteen pounds and her chronic bowel irritability was worse than ever. In order to counter this, she stopped eating many foods. This led to a six-month stretch of bulimia that year. Jane openly discussed that it was very 'fashionable' to regularly make oneself vomit after eating. This was especially true of the women gymnasts, who felt great pressure to keep their tiny physiques.

Throughout college Jane felt exhausted and complained of frequent abdominal, pelvic, and bladder pain. She also started experiencing widespread muscle and joint pains. Her mother had read some studies on fibromyalgia and was convinced that Jane's symptoms matched. When we met, I asked Jane to describe her symptoms:

Last year, I woke up every morning feeling exhausted and sore all over. It felt like I had been working out for hours. I thought I was over-training and our gymnastics coach at school told me to take some time off. But that made me feel worse. I kept pulling muscles in my back and groin. The doctors at the school infirmary could not find anything wrong and told me that I was probably just stressed out. I did not agree. I knew that I had not been eating well so I began to carbohydrate load before my workouts. Then I tried a high-protein diet and also eliminated all wheat and grain. Nothing helped my exhaustion or my abdominal cramps. The pain in my muscles got worse. Just opening a jar hurts my arms. My elbows feel raw. I finally had to quit the gymnastics team. Last month it got so bad that I missed two weeks of school. I had so much pain than I couldn't stand up at times. Every nerve seems tender. My back is in constant spasm. Half the time, I can't tell if it's coming from my stomach or from my back. Everything feels stiff. I feel like I'm eighty years old.

Jane was very petite, 5 feet tall and weighed 98 pounds. For someone as accomplished as she was, Jane appeared very ill at ease when we met. Her eyes rarely looked directly at me. She was constantly fidgeting. The physical examination revealed no evidence of arthritis and no bowel or bladder abnormalities. She did have very tight neck and back muscles. I also found numerous tender points typical of fibromyalgia. Her abdomen was also tight and tender, but the rest of the physical examination and laboratory tests were completely normal.

Jane then described the bladder and pelvic symptoms: *It feels as if I can never fully empty my bladder. As soon as I get comfortable at night I have to run to the lavatory to urinate. I have this constant urgency and feeling of heaviness in the bladder. I was treated twice last year for bladder infections, but the antibiotics worked just for a few weeks. The last two times my doctor arranged microbiological testing of my urine, there was no infection. Then I was sent to a urologist who did a cystoscopy. He said I had interstitial cystitis, but another urologist said that I had an irritable urethra. The medications provided didn't help.*

I've also had irregular periods and terrible menstrual cramps all my life. Two years ago I stopped menstruating for ten months. Since I've started having my period again, the pains have been even worse. A deep discomfort in my groin and pelvic region is always present. My gynaecological examination was okay and no one could tell me what was wrong down there. My boyfriend and I are planning to get married next year. Now, I dread having sex because it has become so painful.

At first Jane was quiet and withdrawn, but as we talked she became more relaxed and lively. When I asked her about her childhood history of bowel trouble, she began to cry. After a few minutes of silence, she told me that her bowel problems began at a time when she was verbally and physically abused by her stepfather. She had never discussed this with her mother for fear that her mother's ulcerative colitis would become much worse. Jane's mother had developed bowel cancer last year, a dreaded complication of ulcerative colitis. This was diagnosed just before Jane developed the muscle, bladder, and pelvic pain.

Jane's chronic gastrointestinal symptoms were typical of IBS. She also had fibromyalgia. Among people with fibromyalgia, 70 percent have IBS. Jane's other symptoms are common in IBS. Of women with IBS, 80 percent report sexual dysfunction, 60 percent complain of chronic fatigue, and 60 percent have bladder irritability. During the first two years of college, Jane had been examined by a number of urologists and gynaecologists. At the age of twenty-one, Jane had already been told that she had fibromyalgia, IBS, CFS, interstitial cystitis, irritable urethral syndrome, and vulvodynia. Cessation of menses, amenorrhoea, may have been a consequence of stress-induced hormonal changes associated with an eating disorder, a common occurrence in young, female athletes. As in fibromyalgia and CFS, medical specialists were trying to find a diagnosis when there was no obvious organic disease.

IBS, just like fibromyalgia, CFS, and migraine, is diagnosed by symptoms. There are no specific physical findings or laboratory tests. The symptoms include a change in bowel habits, with alternating diarrhoea and constipation and abdominal pain. There is often abdominal distention, pain relief with bowel movements, mucus in the stool, and the sensation of incomplete evacuation. And just like in fibromyalgia and CFS, the symptoms used to diagnose IBS were arrived at by a consensus of experts. There have been three different sets of IBS criteria and the most often used is called the Rome criteria. These criteria include continuous or recurrent symptoms of abdominal pain or discomfort that is relieved with defaecation, abdominal pain or discomfort that is associated with a change in frequency of stool or consistency of stool as well as bloating or feeling of abdominal distention.

These symptoms should be present for at least three months before the diagnosis of IBS is entertained. Inflammatory or structural bowel diseases, including ulcerative colitis or Crohn's disease, may also cause these symptoms. Such gastrointestinal diseases must be excluded by taking a careful history and physical examination. Often, a sigmoidoscopy, colonoscopy, or radiologic examination of the bowel will be necessary to exclude structural, neoplastic, or inflammatory bowel diseases.

Symptoms compatible with IBS are present in 10–20 percent of adults. IBS is three times more common in females. IBS is often mild enough that people never seek medical attention. Only a fraction of people in the community who have symptoms of IBS are ever diagnosed or treated. More than 70 percent of gastro-intestinal complaints bringing people to a doctor are never found to have an organic cause. IBS is the most common disorder referred to gastroenterologists. Nevertheless, in the United States the research support for IBS, like for fibromyalgia, has been meager. In 1992, only 0.4 percent of the 140 million dollars for gastro-intestinal research from the National Institutes of Health (NIH) was devoted to IBS or other functional gastrointestinal disorders.

Demographic and psycho-social factors are similar in IBS and fibromyalgia. There is a female predominance. Both are often exacerbated around the menstrual period. The peak age of diag-nosed cases is twenty-five to forty-five. The younger age at diag-nosis may be related in part to a referral bias on doctors' part. Doctors are more likely to diagnose osteoarthritis as a cause of generalized pain in the elderly than fibromyalgia. They are also more likely to diagnose conditions like diverticulitis in the elderly rather than IBS.

Research in IBS suggests important gut and brain connections similar to the muscle and brain connections of fibromyalgia. Enteroendocrine cells in the intestinal lining relay painful stimuli to the spinal cord. Serotonin and other neurohormones regulate these messages. The same pain pathways discussed in fibromyal-gia involving the spinal cord, the brain, and descending modulat-ing fibres are activated in IBS. Central sensitization results in intestinal hyperalgesia and allodynia. Instead of relying on tender-point pain tolerance to demonstrate the muscle hyperalgesia in fibromyalgia, gastroenterologists use rectal balloon or volume distention to reveal the intestinal muscle hypersensitivity in IBS. Imaging studies of the brain's pain centres following rectal distention show greater activation in IBS patients compared with normal subjects.

Infections activate or aggravate IBS, as postulated for fibromyalgia and CFS. Acute viral or bacterial gastroenteritis may trigger IBS. Psycho-social factors interact with biological factors in IBS as in fibromyalgia. Levels of psychological distress were the best predictor for who developed IBS after acute gastrointestinal infections. Physical and emotional abuse, such as Jane had experienced, has been an especially important risk factor for IBS. More than 40 percent of patients attending a gastroenterology clinic for IBS have a history of physical or sexual abuse. Traumatic memories and their flashbacks leave an indelible mark on the brain.

IBS is another example of psyche and body joining forces to cause illness and suffering. The connection of our emotions and our gut has been recognized throughout history. Moses Maimonides, the Jewish physician and scholar, wrote in the twelfth century, 'Humans should strive to have their intestines relaxed all the days of their lives.' In the 1920s and 1930s, IBS patients were characterized as 'constipated, dyspeptic, depressed, introspective, exhausted, emotionally unstable or asthenic. They may be calm externally, but they usually seethe internally, and any strong emotion is likely to affect all those organs that are under the control of the autonomic nerves.'

Psychological factors are part of every disease and every illness. When structural disease is not found, doctors focus on emotional factors. Psycho-social stressors are very important in understanding our response to any chronic illness. The stressor may be simple, such as unhappiness at work or at home. Or more complex factors may be an issue. For some, stress may stem from the distant past, such as an unhappy childhood. Our minds tend to bury our most unpleasant experiences. Jane's repressed emotional and physical trauma left permanent scars. Women who had suffered various forms of childhood abuse were found to have blunted cortisol responses and exaggerated heart rate responses, similar to those described in fibromyalgia patients. A recent report from the Harvard Medical School psychiatric department demonstrated that physical, sexual, or verbal abuse in childhood caused physical changes in the brain. One hemisphere of the brains of children who experienced such abuse was smaller than the other, and the communication between the two hemispheres was impaired. Dr. Martin Teicher commented, 'The brain is fundamentally sculpted by our experiences. Adverse experiences will sculpt our brains in different ways.'

Negative life events are three times more common in people with fibromyalgia and IBS than in healthy individuals. IBS and fibromyalgia patients with a history of chronic emotional trauma report more pain, greater utilization of health-care resources, more surgery, and greater disability than those who did not experience such psychological trauma. Note that the onset of Jane's fibromyalgia and bladder symptoms coincided with her mother's cancer diagnosis.

The treatment of IBS has changed radically. It is now based on the brain–gut connection. The focus is no longer simply to improve gut motility. Prior treatment of IBS consisted of dietary advice, laxative or bulking agents, and antispasmodics. This treatment is of limited success. Pharmacological approaches have now shifted to drugs that reduce intestinal sensation. The antidepressants, such as those used in fibromyalgia and CFS, do this to some degree and are modestly effective in treating IBS. New drugs that block intestinal serotonin receptors have been developed.

A multidisciplinary team approach, as in fibromyalgia, has been the most effective form of therapy for IBS. A non-judgmental relationship with a caring physician is most important in each of these syndromes. I referred Jane to a gastroenterologist who cares for many people with IBS. Some rheumatologists are comfortable seeing lots of patients with poorly understood pain disorders and the same is true with gastroenterologists. He reassured

Jane that the bowel symptoms were treatable although not necessarily curable. Jane kept a diary of foods that aggravated her symptoms. Certain dairy products and vegetables aggravated her bowels, and they were gradually eliminated. More importantly, he discussed her general eating habits and ways to achieve a healthy diet. He focused on her past history of anorexia and bulimia. Food no longer became a central part of Jane's existence.

Jane also used antidiarrhoeal or anti-constipation medications in moderation, depending on which symptoms predominated. When pain, gas, and bloating were especially prominent, antispasmodic agents, such as belladonna or dicyclomine, were helpful. Jane's bowel and fibromyalgia symptoms improved with low doses of tricyclic antidepressants. Whether these medications work as antidepressants, anticholinergics, or analgesics is unclear. However, some of the effects of these medications are clearly independent of their impact on mood.

Jane agreed to see a psychiatric professional to work out the issues of her childhood trauma. At first, this was very difficult for her. Jane's physical and mental well-being both needed attention. The psychiatrist that I work with talked to Jane about the influence of her past and recent severe stress on her symptoms.

Psychologically focused therapies that Jane has tried include psychotherapy and cognitive behavioural therapy. Over the past few years her symptoms have improved, although she still needs to watch what she eats. Her fibromyalgia symptoms are much better and she has resumed exercise, although at a reduced level. Jane still is working with a psychologist, although she no longer takes any antidepressants. Discussions of her abuse during childhood were very traumatic, but proved important. Jane has been more open, less symptomatic, and much more optimistic.

FICTION

- IBS is a structural gastrointestinal disease.

- IBS is caused by food sensitivity and can be cured by dietary changes.

- IBS is caused by bacterial, parasite, and fungal intestinal infections.

- IBS is a stress problem and occurs in Type-A people or people abused during childhood.

FACTS

- IBS is a disorder of gut pain perception. Among people with fibromyalgia, 70 percent suffer from IBS.

- There is no evidence that bacterial or yeast infections cause IBS or that antimicrobial treatment will cure it.

- A history of mood disorders and emotional stress is more common in patients with IBS and fibromyalgia who are treated in specialty clinics compared with community people with similar symptoms.

- Most people with IBS respond well to a combination of medications, dietary changes, and behavioural modification.

7

What Caused It?

CYNTHIA, a thirty-nine-year-old computer programmer, was referred to me by a lawyer to confirm that she had fibromyalgia. She had been involved in two car accidents in the past three years, each time suffering a 'whiplash' neck injury. She recovered and went back to work after the first, although she still experienced neck pain. After the second accident, she developed generalized pain throughout her body and had been out of work ever since.

Cynthia was convinced that the trauma had permanently damaged her spine. She had seen orthopaedic surgeons, neurosurgeons, and chiropractors. Some told her that there was no structural damage. Others diagnosed post-concussive brain damage, carpal tunnel syndrome, wrist tenosynovitis, subluxed cervical vertebrae, cervical and lumbar degenerative disc disease, scoliosis, and nerve entrapment. During the previous eighteen months, Cynthia underwent carpal tunnel surgery as well as cervical spine surgery without any improvement in her pain.

On examination, I found no evidence of spinal or nerve damage. Each of the characteristic fibromyalgia tender points was present.

Cynthia was also complaining of exhaustion, pounding daily headaches, insomnia, depression, abdominal pain, and diarrhoea. I reviewed the X-rays, MRIs, and CAT scans and found no evidence of bone or joint damage. Cynthia's symptoms were compatible with fibromyalgia, muscular headaches, and IBS.

I explained to Cynthia that fibromyalgia may be precipitated by trauma, be it physical or emotional, major or minor. However, her widespread pain was a result of alterations in pain perception rather than from tissue damage. Cynthia disagreed adamantly: *My other doctors told me that my spinal column had been damaged. The MRI was proof of this. The chiropractor showed me how my neck vertebrae had gone out of place on my X-rays. Why would the doctors have done surgery on my neck if there was no permanent damage?* When I interrupted her to suggest that we explore chronic pain mechanisms, Cynthia stormed out of my office with the comment, *you are just like some other doctors who think that I'm making this all up for insurance purposes.*

Two years after a relatively minor 'whiplash' accident, 20 percent of people will complain of chronic neck, shoulder, and upper back pain. They also suffer from headaches, fatigue, sleep disturbances, and sensitivity to light and sounds. Many of my patients with fibromyalgia tell me that their symptoms began after a head or neck injury. A study done by Dr. Dan Buskila and his co-workers in Israel found that fibromyalgia was thirteen times more likely to develop following a neck injury compared with a leg fracture. Is there something peculiar about trauma to the neck region compared with trauma in other parts of the body? Or is the greater incidence of fibromyalgia after such trauma a manifestation of social and cultural phenomena? In Israel, disability and litigation play a minor role in medical issues. Therefore the striking incidence of fibromyalgia following neck injury cannot be simply attributed to potential disability issues. Nevertheless, the role of blame and victimization in people's perception of pain and injury cannot be ignored. People are more likely to blame an accident for their misery if they are the victim rather than if they caused the accident.

Many of my patients became alarmed when they read the front-page article on fibromyalgia in *The Wall Street Journal* (11 November, 1999). The article was titled 'High Hopes: Surgery on the Skull for Chronic Fatigue? Doctors Are Trying It.' Dr. Sam Banner and Ms. Jozan Plaza claimed that brain surgery had cured their fibromyalgia and chronic fatigue: 'Jozan Plaza, a forty-five-year-old Alabama woman, visited Chicago recently to have part of the back of her skull drilled off. Was this a good idea? Ms. Plaza is among the roughly 8 million Americans diagnosed with a condition called fibromyalgia syndrome, which involves widespread muscle pain, sleeplessness, fatigue, and depression. It is poorly understood and controversial. Many doctors aren't convinced it is a disease at all, suspecting in some patients it is really depression with physical manifestations. Patients who are told they have fibromyalgia – or the closely related CFS – are usually just prescribed sleeping pills, antidepressants, and physical therapy. Treating patients with these diagnoses, in short, isn't brain surgery.'

I agreed with their assessment up to that point, but then this news article discussed the contention of two neurosurgeons that a too-tight skull or spinal canal was the cause of fibromyalgia. This spinal narrowing could be congenital, called Chiari syndrome, or acquired from arthritis in the neck. For about $30,000 a case, they were able to relieve the excess pressure on the brain by cutting out pieces of bone in the back of the skull.

I was shocked that such a prestigious newspaper would report such unproven medical concepts. Granted, medical experts such as Dr. Dan Clauw were quoted in *The Wall Street Journal* that such surgery was unlikely to be helpful except in very rare circumstances. Yet, Ms. Plaza's surgeon countered: 'This is like telling the story of the discovery of insulin. You're talking about a completely new insight that has baffled people since the beginning of the modern world.' This Chicago neurosurgeon declared that 100 percent of his patients had improved with this radical new approach. Dr. Michael Rosner, an Alabama neurosurgeon, was the first to suggest that such surgery could help many people with fibromyalgia. He claimed that he had cured hundreds of patients. I began picturing thousands of needless and potentially dangerous brain surgeries performed on people with fibromyalgia.

The hype around this story was ratcheted up a notch when Dr. Tim Johnson interviewed the same two neurosurgeons as well as Sam Banner. These discussions were published in the 12 March, 2000 installment of *20/20*. Barbara Walters introduced the segment with the announcement about 'a radical treatment . . . surgery could be the answer and the cure.' Banner, a family doctor in Alabama, had been felled by chronic fatigue for five years and had to quit his practice. He serendipitously discovered that after Dr. Rosner had operated on patients for Chiari syndrome, many of their symptoms that were similar to Banner's improved. Putting two and two together, Banner ordered an MRI on himself and it revealed spinal cord compression. He was on Dr. Rosner's operating table two days later and Tim Johnson said 'that surgery led to a miraculous recovery for Dr. Banner.' Banner said, 'I went to the chapel and got down on my hands and knees and thanked God.' Dr. Banner then began referring fibromyalgia patients to Dr. Rosner and together they reported that 50 to 80 percent of people with fibromyalgia improved with surgery. Banner also organized a support group and Web site for fibromyalgia and chronic fatigue sufferers. Via these sites and newspaper advertisements, the notion that surgery might be a cure for many people spread like wildfire.

The *20/20* programme did not explain that the symptoms of Chiari malformation and spinal cord compression are very different from the chronic pain and exhaustion that characterize fibromyalgia and CFS. Nor did the programme discuss research that was under way designed to see if these surgeon's observations held up to scientific scrutiny. A study, now completed, compared head and spinal cord MRIs of fibromyalgia patients with those of healthy age- and sex-matched individuals. There was no difference in the prevalence of Chiari malformation or spinal stenosis in the two groups. Nearly 50 percent of completely healthy individuals with no pain and 50 percent of people with fibromyalgia had evidence of some narrowing at the base of the skull. This is reminiscent of the initial enthusiasm in regard to back surgery for herniated lumbar discs. Needless and potentially dangerous surgery was based on overzealous interpretation of new technology such as MRIs.

How can I account for the miraculous results claimed by Dr. Banner and these two neurosurgeons? Some people with fibromyalgia and CFS may also have spinal canal compression. Neurological symptoms such as weakness, abnormal reflexes, vertigo, and paraesthesias might improve if the pressure is relieved. There is also a powerful placebo effect from any intervention as dramatic as surgery. I can state unequivocally that the vast majority of people with fibromyalgia and CFS do not have a surgically curable problem.

Of the more than twenty thousand patients with fibromyalgia that I have examined, physical trauma such as an injury at work or a car accident has been the most common precipitating event. The next most common is an infection, usually described as a viral illness or the flu. Denise told me that her symptoms started with a viral illness: *It felt like I had the flu that never got better.*

Denise's conviction that she had some undetected infection was understandable based on what she had read and heard. One doctor told her that her blood tests proved that she had chronic Epstein-Barr virus infection. Certain physicians and laboratories continue to promote blood tests for Epstein-Barr virus or other chronic viral infections. Such tests are not useful. Denise joined a CFS support group where she was told that scientists were very close to finding an infectious cause of CFS. A number of different viruses including human herpes virus number six initially looked like potential causes. None has been substantiated. Antiviral drugs such as acyclovir have not been useful in treating CFS.

It is possible that medical science will discover that one or more microbes are important in the cause of CFS and fibromyalgia.

Most likely, such an agent will be one of numerous things that can trigger or exacerbate the illness. Viruses or bacteria stress our immune system. They activate neurohormones. That does not mean that the microbe persists in the body (or brain). Denise had read Hillary Johnson's description of CFS as, 'a devastating infectious disease reaching epidemic proportions while government researchers ignore the evidence and the shocking statistics.' Such misconceptions are alarming. A patient with CFS, already racked with uncertainty about their illness, now becomes convinced that they have contracted some rare infection. The controversy about the role of infection is similar to that engulfing chronic Lyme disease.

Lyme disease, so-called because the first reported cases occurred near Lyme, Connecticut, in the United States, is a classic infectious disease like pneumonia and tuberculosis. A microbe enters the skin during a tick bite (which can generally be avoided by staying out of the underbrush or wearing protective clothing). If recognized, a tell-tale skin rash appears at the site of the tick bite. If antibiotics are started at the first signs of a tick bite or the rash, no further problems develop. However, if untreated, the Lyme bacteria, called *Borrelia burgdorfei,* may work its way into joint tissue, causing arthritic pain and swelling. Or it can enter the nervous system and cause paralysis of the seventh cranial nerve (Bell's palsy) or other neurological symptoms. The microbe invades the body and directly damages the tissues. Antibiotics almost always cure Lyme disease even after it affects joints or nerves.

There has been no medical controversy about acute Lyme disease. But there is major controversy regarding the question of a chronic Lyme infection. The leading authorities, including Dr. Allen Steere, who discovered Lyme disease, believe that chronic Lyme disease is rare. Yet some doctors attribute unexplained chronic pain, fatigue, and headaches to chronic Lyme disease. As in the situation with CFS, there has been polarization between the academic community and certain patient-advocate groups. These groups and their doctor supporters argue that the Lyme bacteria routinely hide deep within cells of the body, which are relatively inaccessible to routine antibiotic therapy. There is no evidence for this. Dr. Steere and other scientists have stressed that the mis-diagnoses and anxiety about Lyme disease have become more of a problem than Lyme disease itself.

Some patients do remain ill long after Lyme infection has seem-ingly been eradicated. Such was the situation with Betsy, who con-sulted me in 1998 after suffering from muscle and joint pain and persistent fatigue for three years. In the spring of 1995, while on holiday in northern New England, in the United States, she devel-oped a large, circular rash on her right thigh. Although she did not remember a tick bite, she had been walking through a marsh where Lyme disease had been reported. During the next few days, Betsy had run a low-grade fever, felt very tired and achy, and had a sore right knee. She saw her family doctor, who told her that the rash was characteristic of that seen in the earliest stages of Lyme disease. A blood test demonstrated antibodies that confirmed recent Lyme infection. The doctor prescribed a two-week course of antibiotics, the standard therapy for recently acquired Lyme disease.

During the next few weeks, Betsy gradually felt better. Her fever and skin rash disappeared and never returned. However, after six months, the fatigue returned. She also began to experience muscle and joint pains, dizziness, mental confusion, and severe headaches.

A specialist was consulted who told Betsy that he suspected spread of Lyme disease to the central nervous system. To deter-mine whether there were bacteria in the brain and spinal fluid, Betsy underwent two spinal taps, an EEG, a brain and spinal cord MRI, and multiple blood tests. All results were normal, but he told Betsy that she had chronic Lyme infection of the nervous sys-tem. She was placed on a month-long course of intravenous antibiotics. During that month, she felt slightly more energetic, but over the next year the muscle pains, fatigue, headaches, and cognitive disturbances persisted. In 1997, she had another four-week trial of a different and 'stronger' antibiotic. She noted no improvement.

When I evaluated Betsy, she complained of severe fatigue and muscle pain. Her physical examination was unremarkable except for extreme tenderness over the fibromyalgia 'tender points.' Her neurological examination was normal. The blood tests demonstrated that she had been infected with the Lyme bacteria in the past, but very sensitive tests found no evidence for persistent, active Lyme infection. I told Betsy that she had fibromyalgia and CFS, which might have been triggered by the Lyme infection. The original Lyme infection had been eradicated by antibiotics. I treated her with a low dose of amitriptyline at bedtime which helped her to sleep better and improved her muscle pain. During the next six months, she gradually felt less exhaustion, and the headaches and dizziness disappeared. She was relieved to be told that her brain had not been invaded by the Lyme bacteria.

An even more common situation involves patients who believe that they have Lyme disease, but in fact never did. Last year, Veronica came to see me to determine whether she did or did not have Lyme disease. She told me: *In December I had a sore throat and fever of a 103 degrees that lasted for three days. My family doctor put me on antibiotics and I began to feel better. Four days after that I developed a very itchy rash on my legs and my back. My doctor thought I might be allergic to the antibiotic and discontinued it and put me on oral tetracycline. Then I began getting aches and pains all over my body. Over the next three months I felt washed out and ached all over. All my blood tests were normal and I went on and off antibiotics for the next few months. Finally an infectious disease specialist saw me. He obtained a blood test and told me that I probably had Lyme disease. When I spoke to him I remembered that I had been bitten by something the summer before. I don't recall any skin rash. Now I have been on intravenous or oral antibiotics for the past six months. I still feel lousy.*

When I examined Veronica, I found no evidence of any rash or arthritis. I did a careful neurological examination, which was normal. The rest of her examination was unremarkable except that I found muscle tenderness in the typical fibromyalgia locations. I told Veronica that this was not Lyme disease. She had fibromyalgia.

Most people who have been treated with antibiotics for suspected Lyme disease *without improvement* probably never had Lyme disease at all. They more likely had fibromyalgia and chronic fatigue, which are much more common than Lyme disease. Even where Lyme disease is endemic, as in New England, fewer than .01 percent of the population (one in ten thousand) ever develop the disease. In contrast, 5 percent of the population have fibromyalgia and chronic fatigue.

That means that fibromyalgia and CFS are five hundred times more common than Lyme disease. And the blood tests for Lyme disease can be just as misleading as they are in CFS. People who live in tick-infested areas often develop antibodies against the Lyme bacteria, but never get sick. In such people, a 'false positive' antibody test result may lead to antibiotic treatment for Lyme disease that is useless and ignores the real problem. To avoid this mistake, doctors should perform Lyme antibody tests only in patients with signs and symptoms that are clinically suggestive of Lyme disease.

With the media attention and scare about Lyme disease, people worry that their everyday aches and fatigue may be caused by undetected Lyme disease. A prominent doctor wrote: 'Lots of people who are stressed out or who have chronic fatigue syndrome are picking Lyme disease and finding physicians to be willing accomplices, willing to treat them with expensive, even experimental antibiotics, in the absence of real proof that they have Lyme disease. Not surprisingly, they don't get better.' A *New York Times Magazine* feature from 8 July, 2001, entitled 'Stalking Doctor Steere' described the 'growing number of patient advocacy groups and physicians who argued that chronic Lyme disease had become a full-scale epidemic, a modern-day plague crippling thousands of Americans. As the world's foremost expert on the illness, however, Steere did not believe many of them had Lyme disease at all, but something else – chronic fatigue or mental illness or fibromyalgia – and he had refused to treat them with antibiotics . . . hordes of patients had started to stalk him. They depicted him in the media as a demon, worse than the spirochetes, the tick-borne bacteria that they claimed inhabited their bodies and that, because of his restrictive diagnosis, they could not eliminate.' It took me months to convince Veronica that she had fibromyalgia, not Lyme disease.

Denise was diagnosed with multiple chemical sensitivity syndrome by a specialist called a clinical ecologist. Ecologists have popularized supposed 'environmental illnesses' such as the candidiasis hypersensitivity syndrome (popularly known as 'The Yeast Connection'), total allergy syndrome, and chemically induced immune dysregulation. They contend that many illnesses – from cancer to CFS – are caused by chemicals in the air that we breathe or the food that we eat. They postulate that 'environmental illnesses' overwhelm the immune system of susceptible individuals who cannot adapt to society's profusion of synthetic chemicals. They perform tests purported to reveal that person's specific sensitivities. These substances are then gradually eliminated from the person's diet or surroundings.

However, there is no scientific evidence that dietary or environmental substances *cause* syndromes like CFS and fibromyalgia. It can be difficult to discount the notion that chemicals in our environment cause illnesses. We have all experienced distress when exposed to noxious irritants such as smoke, car exhaust fumes, ammonia, pesticides, paint, and glue. We can all get sick from such compounds. But these reactions rarely cause chronic health problems. I couldn't totally discount that some substance in Denise's workplace might have been a factor in her becoming sick yet there is no evidence that environmental toxins are causes of chronic illness like fibromyalgia or CFS. Many of the blood, urine, and skin tests performed for chemical sensitivities are not scientifically validated. Positive results are largely uninterpretable. The public is inundated with these quasi-scientific explanations and rarely hears the scientific evidence against such unfounded theories.

Human beings tend to attribute their medical illnesses to circumstances that are beyond themselves. If patients with CFS or fibromyalgia understand that their illness is not necessarily 'caused' by a hidden infection or undiscovered toxin, they will feel less like victims and more in control. Infectious agents, environmental toxins, and physical trauma play important roles in fibromyalgia and CFS. They contribute to most chronic illness. They are no more or less factors in how we experience illness than our genes, our childhood, and our culture.

FICTION

- **Fibromyalgia and CFS are caused by compression of the spinal cord and brain and may be surgically corrected.**

- **Multiple chemical sensitivity and sick building syndromes are specific illnesses caused by toxic substances.**

- **Chronic Lyme disease is very common and usually unrecognized. Long-term antibiotic treatment is required.**

- **Most chronic illnesses are caused by microbes or environmental toxins.**

- **You can't get better until you know why you are ill.**

FACTS

- Most chronic illnesses are not caused by a single disease mechanism.

- Physical trauma and infections may play a role in triggering or exacerbating chronic illness.

- Many commercial tests said to demonstrate associations of illnesses like fibromyalgia or CFS with an infection or a chemical substance are not reliable.

- Many people who are diagnosed with a chronic infection related to possible Lyme disease or Epstein-Barr virus disease have fibromyalgia and CFS.

- Chronic illnesses have multiple contributing factors, some inside of us, some outside of us.

- We should concentrate on treating the symptoms of chronic illness, not searching for a cause.

8

Is It All in My Head?

VIRGINIA was referred to me by a colleague from Atlanta, Georgia. He had been perplexed by her multiple medical symptoms. Virginia was sixty-five-years old when she and her husband, Alan, came to my consulting room in the spring of 1997. I immediately became wary when Virginia introduced herself with the exclamation, *Dr. Goldenberg, you are my last hope. If you don't find out what is wrong, I don't know what I'll do. My doctors think I'm a hypochondriac, but they don't know what I feel.*

I'm never comfortable with being anyone's 'last hope.' My unease grew when Alan dragged in a very large suitcase stuffed with Virginia's medical records. Virginia had already seen many medical specialists throughout the United States.

Virginia had painstakingly chronicled her medical history. Each of six large, loose-leaf folders was devoted to one of her primary medical disorders. The first folder was labeled 'My stomach and bowel disease.' The other folders were titled: 'Joint and muscle pain,' 'Heart disease,' 'Headaches and memory loss,' 'Neurological disease,' and 'Immunological problems.' Each folder had at least five sub-sections. Dates of her multiple different doctor appointments and hospitalizations were indexed and then cross-referenced. I told Virginia that it would take me hours, but that I would review her medical records. I suggested that she first tell me about herself.

She responded by describing the onset of her first medical symptoms when she was a young girl. I stopped her in mid-sentence and told her that I wanted to first hear about her life, apart from her illness. Virginia was taken aback. Her life and her self-identity had revolved around her sickness. I reassured Virginia that I would listen to her medical complaints, but that I also wanted to understand her as a person, not just as a patient. Somewhat reluctantly, she began to tell me about her childhood.

Virginia grew up in a suburb, west of Atlanta, Georgia, in the southern United States, the daughter of a very well-known and respected general surgeon. She was the youngest of four children, and two of her older brothers were doctors. Virginia, the youngest child and only girl, had been pampered. She felt close to her brothers, not her parents. She remembered: *We were well off – although I wouldn't say we were rich. Our house had a maid and a cook and I had a nanny. She took care of me and I only saw my mother 'by appointment.' Everything was much more formal in those days. We had a three-course meal every night and my father always wore a tie and jacket to dinner.*

Our routine at home revolved around my father's busy schedule. At dinner, the telephone sat poised next to him and dinner was often interrupted by calls from patients or other doctors. We would all have to be quiet. I remember feeling a sense of pride that he was so important, but also some resentment that everything centred around his schedule. Everyone in our town knew my father and always told me what a brilliant and wonderful man he was. I never saw much of him during the week, although he would always sit and talk to me on Sunday mornings. He would read me stories. When I was older, we would discuss books or my school-work or boys. Every summer, my father would take a holiday for a full month and our whole family would go somewhere special. We took the maid, the cook, and the nanny, and would go to a ranch out West or to a fishing lodge in the Maine woods.

Virginia then described how 'sickly' she had been throughout her childhood: *I missed school a lot because of headaches and stomach aches. I remember being out most of the year during third grade. My father thought that I might have had a mild case of polio. So they kept me at home that winter. After that, I never felt well. I couldn't keep up with the other kids during school. My legs always hurt and felt like they were giving out. We went to see a lot of specialists, one who thought it might be rheumatic fever. But, after a while, the doctors concluded that it was 'growing pains.'*

Virginia then recounted her initial hospitalization: *I was in my first year at college. I remember feeling totally exhausted and I couldn't sleep. I started getting awful feelings in my arms and legs – they would get cold and then numb. My headaches were terrible, and I felt sick all the time. Finally I was hospitalized at the university health service, but they couldn't find out what was wrong. My father came to get me and he told me that I had an ulcer. I thought only older people got ulcers. Dad brought me to his hospital in Atlanta, where I was treated for the ulcer for two weeks. But I have had stomach trouble ever since.*

Virginia went on to describe the next twenty years of her persistent medical problems. The stomach pains, cramps, and constipation or diarrhoea persisted. She had three operations, first for an ulcer at the age of thirty, then at thirty-five her gall bladder was removed. At forty-eight she had a further operation to correct intestinal adhesions. Each surgery made her pain decrease for a few months, but then all of her gastrointestinal symptoms returned. Her headaches gradually got worse, and she took codeine or oxycodone frequently.

Around the age of forty, she began to experience severe, unrelenting numbness in her arms and legs. She became weak and would fall with no warning. During the next fifteen years, she was hospitalized twelve times in search of the cause of her pain, weakness, and numbness. At the age of fifty-six she was hospitalized twice for chest pain, initially felt to be angina or a minor heart attack. No heart disease was found. Her cardiologist told her that he suspected the pain was from costochondritis, inflammation of the chest muscles.

Virginia flew all over the country in search of a diagnosis for her multiple ailments. She went to the Mayo Clinic twice, the Lahey Clinic in Boston, and visited four neurologists in New York and at Duke Medical Center. Two neurologists diagnosed possible multiple sclerosis, but the two other neurologists disagreed. She was very upset when she consulted a world-famous neurologist in New York: *He told me that all my pain and other medical problems were in my head. The neurologist implied that I was hysterical and making up these symptoms for attention. He asked me to see a psychiatrist, who told me that I was depressed. Of course I was depressed after all the pain and suffering. Who wouldn't be? But how could he think that my pain and weakness weren't real? I refused to see any new doctors after that.*

During the 1990s, Virginia's health continued to deteriorate. She resorted to using a Zimmer frame or a cane to get around. Alan, a successful businessman, stayed home much of each week to take care of her. At the time of her appointment, Virginia was taking nine different medications every day, three for her heart, three for 'nerve pain,' and three different 'tranquillizers.' I asked Virginia to describe her leg pain to me: *The pain is always there. At times, when I move around or start to walk, it feels like a hot poker running down my leg into my foot. The chest pain is a heavy, dull pressure over my sternum. When I first began getting the chest pain in my fifties, I would become very anxious and think I was having a heart attack. Now, the chest pains aren't as frightening. But the leg pain is terrible – nothing helps it. Even when the leg pain lets up, my balance is off, and I will fall on my face if I try to walk too much. Lately, I've remained in bed for most of the day.*

I reviewed the extensive medical reports on Virginia. Every conceivable neurological, orthopaedic, gastrointestinal, and cardiac test had been done on her during the past twenty years. She had six different MRIs, four CAT scans, even two spinal taps. Nothing was found. Her physical examination was unremarkable except for the typical fibromyalgia tender points. It was therefore reasonable to conclude that her numerous unexplained medical symptoms were all part of the fibromyalgia complex. The widespread muscle pain, the burning and numbness in her extremities, and the chronic headaches and chronic exhaustion all fit the bill. The non-cardiac chest pain and the non-ulcer dyspepsia are common in fibromyalgia.

What was different with Virginia was the severity of each of her many symptoms. When I applied moderate pressure to any muscle, she reacted violently. Such dramatic pain response always alerts doctors to the emotional aspects of pain. About 10 percent of patients with fibromyalgia exhibit such extreme reaction to light touching anywhere on their bodies. Like Virginia, these patients report hyperirritability to everything around them. They can't tolerate light, noise, or smells. Some of these patients won't even let me examine them. With the histrionic nature of her symptoms, no wonder doctors thought Virginia was hysterical.

Strangely, we almost never accuse men of being hysterical. In fact, the word *hysteria* derives from the Greek word *hystera*, which means 'uterus.' In ancient medical lore, hysteria was thought to be caused by the uterus travelling around the body. Plato wrote: 'The womb is an animal which longs to generate children. When it remains barren too long after puberty, it is distressed and sorely disturbed, and straying about in the body and cutting off the passages of the breath, it impedes respiration and brings the sufferer into the extremist anguish and provokes all manner of diseases besides.' Current medical jargon includes *globus hystericus,* referring to the psychogenic choking sensations described by Plato.

Doctors and scientists have always struggled with understanding medical symptoms when no objective disease is present. Hysteria is considered to be an emotional disorder. In 1667, Dr. Thomas Willis, the father of neurology, cautioned, 'As we have shown before, the passions vulgarly called "hysterical" do not always proceed from the womb, but often from the head being affected.' After Freud, psychological and psychosexual explanations for hysterical personalities became the province of psychiatrists.

A gender bias also plays a part in debates about the emotional components of chronic illnesses. Fibromyalgia, CFS, migraine, IBS, and depression are all more common in women than in men. Some doctors and many people in our society believe that women react more emotionally to stress. In a male-dominated society, female problems are easily brushed aside. Female sickliness and psychosexual influences characterize the history of hysteria. I often hear from my male colleagues that women with fibromyalgia just need a 'stiff upper lip.'

Hysteria, psychosomatic, hypochondriasis, somatization, and functional illness are terms used when medical symptoms can't be explained by organic disease. Hypochondriasis has been defined as an excess or unjustified fear or belief in disease. The terms *hysteria* and *hypochondriasis* have largely been replaced in current psychiatric jargon by 'somatization,' the conversion of psychological distress into physical symptoms. Each of these labels describes people like Virginia, who are convinced that they are suffering from a physical disease when none can be found. They reject any notion that their symptoms are emotionally based. Whether called hysterics, hypochondriacs, or somatizers, somatically focused people are thought to magnify their physical symptoms. Somatization is different from malingering. Rather than faking an illness, the somatizing patient is expressing real symptoms that he or she is convinced have an organic basis. Somatization is not a disease. It simply means that a person is excessively concerned about their symptoms. Exaggerated health concerns are almost unavoidable in illnesses such as fibromyalgia. When the diagnosis is elusive people focus more on their bodies and fear the worst.

Illness labels like 'hypochondriasis' and 'psychosomatic' are pejorative, implying that the physical symptoms are imaginary. These terms should be discarded. The current, more appropriate term for an illness that lacks objective findings is a 'functional syndrome.' This implies that abnormalities in the physical functioning of the body exist, but they can't be explained by structural changes.

It is difficult to determine whether physical symptoms are part or purely psychologically driven. Virginia's chest pain resulted in numerous visits to hospital emergency departments and a number of hospitalizations. Both she and her doctors thought that she might be having a heart attack. She described a typical bout: *The pain often woke me during the night quite suddenly. It felt like someone was sitting on my chest. My breathing would become laboured and I would get cold and clammy. I could feel my heart racing. When I would lie down, my pulse would be pounding in my ear so hard that my head moved.*

There are clues that a psychological source may be generating physical ailments. Virginia had complained of a vast array of medical problems for many years. The finest diagnosticians in the land were not able to find a disease that caused her headaches, stomach pains, and chest pains. Virginia's descriptions of her pain were dramatic. She told me that her leg pain 'felt like a hot poker' and that her headaches 'felt like my head was exploding.' Such theatrical responses are common in psychologically charged illnesses. Yet, despite her vivid pain descriptive narratives, Virginia seemed to be emotionally blunted. Instead of demonstrating grief, frustration, fear, or unhappiness, her emotions were all channelled into the physical symptoms.

Excess health concerns are not solely the province of hypochondriacs. We all have times when we get more worried and exaggerate our health concerns. The more that we focus on our body, the more that new symptoms crop up. Then we see doctors over and over. It is easier to imagine that there is something wrong with the organs of our body than to chip away at potential stressors in our emotional lives. We have become a society of worried well. At least two-thirds of all visits to general practitioners are for non-sickness. In general practice, more than 50 percent of complaints are never found to have an organic basis.

Much of this excess illness worry is generated by the medical profession. Most doctors are more skilled and more comfortable at searching for physical rather than for emotional ailments. Therefore, blood is drawn, X-rays are taken, and specialists are consulted. Our patients get the message that physical complaints receive more respect and attention than emotional ones. Dr. Arthur Barsky, a Harvard psychiatrist, has written about the 'paradox of health,' a growing preoccupation with sickness and disability despite improvement in our health status. Daily life stresses and experiences are framed in a medical rather than a psychosocial context. Human beings have become increasingly convinced that any distress and discomfort is abnormal and should be relieved. Universal symptoms such as fatigue, headaches, backaches, rashes, dizziness, and diarrhoea are elevated to the status of a disease. This has been termed *medicalization*. The media bombards us with the latest headache and back pain panacea. Healthcare providers and members of industry reap benefits from this medicalization of everyday complaints.

Dr. Barsky and another psychiatrist, Dr. Edward Shorter, have written extensively about the social and cultural factors promoting the medicalization of symptoms. Barsky attributes much of this to the rising anti-scientific sentiment in society. There is a decline in the authority and prestige of doctors. A simple pat on the back and reassurance no longer alleviate people's anxiety. The wealth of unfiltered media and Internet information spreads rumours and anecdotes. Shorter has called these non-disease states 'bizarre new illness attributions, held as articles of faith by the patients, but supported neither by scientific evidence nor the patina of plausibility.'

Fibromyalgia and CFS are by their definition functional disorders. There is no objective physical basis for the characteristic symptoms. This does not mean that people with fibromyalgia are hysterical or hypochondriacs. Unfortunately, the functional or psychosomatic label is usually interpreted as all psychological. Dr. John Sarno, author of a popular book on back pain, links functional syndromes to emotional trauma, especially repressed unconscious rage. These run the gamut from fibromyalgia to myofascial pain syndrome, carpal tunnel syndrome, reflex sympathetic dystrophy, CFS, temporomandibular joint syndrome, headaches, IBS, allergies, peptic ulcer disease, and oesophageal reflux. Criticizing the current focus on the biology of the brain, Sarno comments, 'In my experience backache, stomach ache, and headache are almost always psychologically induced. Rejection of the role of unconscious emotional phenomena is part of the current trend to bash Freud. Contemporary psychiatry prefers to use drugs and behavioral techniques to treat patients rather than get involved in the messy business of exploring the person's unconscious.' Sarno concludes that since these symptoms are emotionally driven, they can be abolished by a person's own free will.

These doctors equate non-organic illness with emotionally exaggerated illness. Medicine often changes its viewpoint regarding the organic causes of illnesses. For most of the past century, peptic ulcer disease was considered to be largely related to stress. The Type-A personality was predisposed to ulcers. We now recognize that a bacterium, called *H. pylori,* is an important cause of stomach ulcers. That doesn't mean that stress is no longer a factor. Migraine is now considered to have a biological rather than a psychogenic basis. However, ignoring the role of stress in migraine is a costly oversight. The physiological changes in fibromyalgia, CFS, and IBS suggest that in the near future these illnesses will also have greater biological acceptability.

Doctors, whether internal medicine specialists or psychiatrists, are usually very frustrated when treating patients such as Virginia. A person's persistent preoccupation with multiple, unexplained physical symptoms is a doctor's worst nightmare. Dr. Barsky cautioned that people with fibromyalgia, 'become trapped in the belief that their symptoms are due to disease, with future expectations of debility and doom. This enhances their vigilance about their body, and thus the intensity of their symptoms.'

Medicines often don't work. Counselling is often rejected or of little utility. Virginia, like most somatically focused people, saw many doctors all over the country, but never received a firm disease diagnosis. She was probed, prodded, and cut open. Then she was brushed off or lectured to.

Doctors assume that people like Virginia exaggerate their physical symptoms and use their sick role in order to gain attention. Virginia, like the vast majority of people with fibromyalgia, was neither malingering nor did she want to be ill. In all probability, her childhood and family experiences created an environment that fostered excess somatic concerns. Her mother was cold and aloof. Professionally and personally, Virginia's father was precise, demanding, and intense. Disease could be excised or expunged. Virginia had felt closest to her father during her own childhood illnesses. It was then that he became a doting, concerned father, more responsive to her than to his patients. After forty years of assuming the 'sick role,' both as a daughter and as a wife, counselling or psychotherapy would likely have little impact on such an emotional investment.

Genetic factors are as important as environmental factors in determining any person's preoccupation with bodily symptoms. Here, too, nature and nurturing combine. Based on research in twins, it was found that one-third of excess somatic concern was related to specific genetic differences in people. The 'set points' for how we respond to stress and pain can be permanently altered by early life trauma.

The vast majority of people with fibromyalgia are not somatizers or hypochondriacs. However, it is difficult for patients who suffer the uncertainties of fibromyalgia to not worry too much or complain too loudly when their doctors find nothing wrong. People with fibromyalgia are looked on sceptically; they must prove that they have a 'real illness.' Virginia had kept looking for verification that she was ill. Each new expert gave her hope that she would be labelled with a 'real' disease and then cared for. Each time Virginia would be dismissed as 'not sick.'

Gradually, with counselling and attention, Virginia's symptoms improved. The psychiatrist that I work with and I both talked frankly with Virginia about her life-long sick role. This did not mean that her symptoms were imaginary. It did mean that she needed to focus less on her illnesses and more on her health. Frequent visits were required before she was willing to explore in greater depth the family dynamics that played such an important role in her illness. She also accepted my suggestion to try a low dose of a serotonin reuptake inhibitor. This decreased her fibromyalgia symptoms and made her feel less overwhelmed. Gradually her symptoms diminished.

We all must guard against equating *unexplained* physical symptoms with *exaggerated* physical symptoms. We can't easily see or accurately measure the pain and suffering of fibromyalgia, CFS, migraine, and depression. Nevertheless, it is every bit as real as the pain experienced from an injury or inflammation.

FICTION

- **Fibromyalgia is a somatization disorder; people told that they have fibromyalgia, CFS, or IBS are hypochondriacs.**

- **Most common disorders such as fibromyalgia, headaches, and CFS are caused by repressed emotional rage.**

- **You can cure yourself of these symptoms only if you accept their emotional basis.**

FACTS

- Illnesses such as fibromyalgia and CFS have no structural basis, but physiological changes in function are present. These illnesses are appropriately called 'functional syndromes.'

- Most chronic illnesses are shaped by biological, emotional, and cultural factors.

- Excess somatic concern is prominent when physical symptoms are unexplained. We must guard against exaggerated fears about our health.

9

Am I Just Depressed?

SARAH came to see me for the first time a few years ago. She was forty-two, but reported a long history of generalized muscle pain and fatigue. Tall, bohemian-appearing, and dressed in a flowing gown with a matching cape, she made a dramatic arrival at my office. Sarah seemed disorganized as she fumbled anxiously through her records and reports. Her penetrating, blue eyes reflected sadness. Worry lines were etched deeply in her brow.

She explained that muscle and joint pain had bothered her for years. During her late twenties, she went to numerous doctors, none of whom found anything wrong. She commented: *I decided that I would just learn to live with all the pain. I thought that it was normal to feel sore and to ache all of the time.*

When I examined Sarah, the fibromyalgia sites were very tender in her neck, shoulders, chest wall, and back. The rest of her general physical examination and neurological examinations were normal. Sarah seemed quite depressed. I asked her to tell me more about her life.

Sarah grew up in a middle-class town on the outskirts of

Boston. She described her own childhood and early adult years as happy but 'stressful.' Sarah told me: *Growing up, I always demanded a lot of myself. Although I was popular, I didn't have many close friends. When I was about fifteen, I started experiencing a lot of highs and lows. During the highs, I had limitless energy. I could stay up all night and never feel tired. That's when I began to paint and write poetry. But during the lows, I felt exhausted and blue. My mother also had a lot of mood swings, so I thought it was inherited. And since my blue periods would usually last only a day or two, I wasn't worried.*

My father wrote film reviews for a big-city newspaper. We would see every foreign and American film before they were released. We got along well, but I always wanted to impress him. Sometimes he would put my ideas in his column. He liked his job, but he had always wanted to write a serious novel. After ten years of work on his 'opus,' Dad was devastated when he couldn't get it published.

In college, my passion for painting grew. I studied art and poetry and loved to do both. I was ecstatic when I sold my first few paintings. I felt indestructible. I could go days with just a couple hours of sleep and paint all night long. I skipped most of my classes and dropped out of college in my second year to concentrate on my career as an artist. My boyfriend and I moved to New York City and we rented a loft in the Village. During the next five years we travelled all over the world. We got married and my daughter Meredith was born. Then everything fell apart, including our marriage. After five years of bickering and unhappiness, we split up.

That was about the time that I really got depressed. There were many days when I could not get out of bed. I lost my appetite and had to force myself to eat. The muscle pains became intolerable. After a while, I couldn't even paint or write. My arms and neck were so weak and ached so much that I couldn't hold the paintbrush. It was impossible to focus or concentrate on my work. I felt restless and agitated all the time. When I was able to paint, all of the colours looked grey. Simple things like shopping for food were overwhelming. My friends stopped coming over or phoning because I ignored them.

A good friend convinced me to see her psychiatrist. He quickly concluded that I was depressed. I was given Prozac but I never took it. I was very reluctant to take any medication. When I was twenty-five, I had lived for one year at an artist's colony in Sausalito, California. One of the gurus there was vehemently opposed to any drugs that 'poison our brains and dull our creativity.' But I got more and more depressed. Every part of me was aching. For two months, I never left my apartment. Meredith went to live with my mum after I convinced my family that I had a deadline to finish a new poetry book. I couldn't stand to be with anyone. A number of times I considered suicide. It was all planned out. If it wasn't for Meredith, I'm sure I would have done it.

One day I made myself go to the supermarket to do some shopping. It was a beautiful autumn day, but it felt like the middle of winter to me. At the supermarket, I was so confused that I couldn't remember what I was doing or why I was there. At the checkout, I couldn't remember how to use my credit card. The cashier got upset that I was holding up the queue. Then I began screaming back at him and collapsed in a heap of uncontrollable sobs. My mother fetched me and signed me into a psychiatric ward. With various antidepressants, anti-anxiety drugs, and counselling, I gradually felt better.

During the past two years I have been on and off medications. I don't feel suicidal any more, but I still get depressed. And I am always exhausted. The pain in my neck and shoulders and back never goes away. The exhaustion feels different than when I was so depressed. It feels more physical. They keep changing my medication but nothing lasts.

Sarah had a life-long history of depression, which at times was bipolar (manic-depressive) in nature. Just as in fibromyalgia and CFS, the diagnosis of depression is based on the clinical symptoms. There are no physical findings or laboratory tests to confirm the diagnosis. Current diagnostic classification of clinical depression requires five of the following nine symptoms: loss of interest in pleasurable activities, sleep disturbances, guilt, loss of energy, concentration problems, appetite loss, agitation, suicidal thoughts, and depressed mood. Obviously, many of these symptoms overlap with those of fibromyalgia and CFS. Generalized muscle pain, headaches, and bowel irritability are also common with depression.

At some time in their lives, 10–20 percent of Americans will have an episode of major depression. Twice as many women as men are diagnosed with depression. For many, depression is recurrent. If you have one bout of depression, there is a 50 percent likelihood of getting another bout. For some, depression is chronic.

Depression takes a huge toll on our health and well being. Clinical depression accounts for more days lost from work than arthritis, diabetes, chronic lung disease, or hypertension. Depression costs the United States $50 billion a year. Depressed people can't get on with life, can't 'put one foot in front of the other.' Often they can't work. Many resort to illicit drugs. As with Sarah, marriages collapse. Up to 15 percent of untreated depressed people will kill themselves. In 1995, 20 percent of high school students considered suicide and 8 percent actually made an attempt. Suicide is even more prevalent in elderly, depressed people.

Sarah was clinically depressed. She also had typical fibromyalgia symptoms. Both had been present for years. She asked me which had come first, but I couldn't tell her. Furthermore, it did not matter. Both needed to be treated.

At the time of diagnosis, 30 to 40 percent of fibromyalgia patients are depressed or have significant anxiety. There is an even greater past history of depression in people with fibromyalgia. More than 70 percent of fibromyalgia patients have experienced at least one bout of depression in their lives. This is significantly higher than the general population, and it is also higher than in rheumatoid arthritis or other chronic pain disorders.

Sleep disturbances are as prominent in depression as in fibromyalgia and CFS. However, the sleep abnormalities differ.

Most depressed patients have a long sleep latency, which is the time required to fall into deep sleep. Depression alters the normal sleep-circadian rhythm. In fact, depression sometimes improves with 'realignment' by deliberate sleep deprivation. These sleep rhythm alterations are not found in fibromyalgia.

Depression causes a penetrating physical and emotional pain that is impossible to describe. Authors who have been depressed grope for words to characterize the pain of depression. In *Darkness Visible*, William Styron wrote: 'I was feeling in my mind a sensation close to, but indescribably different from, actual pain. . . . That the word "indescribable" should present itself is not fortuitous, since it has to be emphasized that if pain were readily describable, most of the countless sufferers from this ancient affliction would have been able to confidently depict for their friends and loved ones (even their physicians) some of the actual dimensions of their torment. . . . For myself, the pain is most closely connected to drowning or suffocation – but even those images are off the mark.'

People don't recognize that depression unleashes a Pandora's box of physical symptoms. Fatigue, abdominal pain, muscle pain, and headaches accompany depression. Forgetfulness and concentration problems are prominent in depression.

Sarah became distraught when I explained that her physical symptoms were connected to depression. She told me: *Before, I thought that my physical symptoms were from fibromyalgia. Now you tell me that even those are because I'm depressed. I hate to think that all of my pain is emotional. I feel guilty about it.*

Sarah could deal better with physical illness because, '*it was beyond my control.*' But, for her, depression was a character flaw. I was well aware of her dilemma. I had never accepted the notion that my own headaches, sleep disturbances, and fatigue were interconnected with and aggravated by depression and anxiety. After all, my recurrent sinus infections were a logical 'physical' explanation for my headaches and exhaustion. If we do have a 'physical illness' we tell ourselves that we are down and irritable because of the medical disease. This is often termed a 'reactive depression.'

When we are physically ill, any co-existing depression is conveniently overlooked and thus untreated. Two-thirds of doctors miss the presence of depression in patients with other medical problems. Clinical depression is present in 50 percent of people after a heart attack, a stroke, or with cancer. After a heart attack, 75 percent remain depressed for as long as a year. During that year, depression is an independent risk factor for death. Depression adds to the burden of any disease and worsens the outcome.

Doctors are often judgmental regarding the 'appropriateness' of depression occuring during another illness. A colleague said that depression is natural, meaning appropriate and acceptable, in his patients with crippling rheumatoid arthritis or cancer. In 'less severe' problems, like fibromyalgia, CFS, or headaches, he is not as accepting. Depression is a serious illness whether present by itself or with another illness. To let it go untreated causes tragic harm and may cause death. Less than one-half of Americans with major depression are being treated.

Why do most of us hide the illness of depression? The very notion that we are suffering from depression or severe anxiety, rather than a 'physical disorder,' places a whole layer of obstacles in the path of becoming healthy again. Even the medically sophisticated person knows that, however enlightened his or her own view of depression is, many people will not understand. Our society's continuing failure to accept mood disturbances as a 'legitimate' illness promotes feelings of guilt and shame. Sarah felt guilty for '*bringing this on myself.*'

The psychiatric profession is partly to blame for the shroud of secrecy and shame that cloaks mental illness. Psychiatric treatment has been behind closed (and often locked) doors. In the name of protecting one's privacy, psychiatric diagnoses or information have been largely inaccessible. We fear that anyone, especially our employers or insurers, will learn that we have a psychiatric illness. Secrecy leads to lack of understanding.

Until recently, psychiatry has focused on the emotional aspects of illness. Psychoanalysis, an in-depth, intense evaluation of one's self, dominated the field. Medical sciences, grounded in biology, looked askance at 'shrinks.' The notion that depression is a biological disorder is relatively recent. Before the eighteenth century, the mentally ill were thought to be possessed by demons. They were isolated in asylums. At the dawn of medical enlightenment, psychiatry was initially seen as an offshoot of neurology.

The father figure of psychiatry and psychotherapy, Sigmund Freud, began his career as a neurologist. He initially believed that mental illness was largely related to observable physiological phenomena. However, Freud gradually abandoned such a biological theory and adopted a strictly psychological interpretation of depression. Neurology and psychiatry split into separate disciplines. Neurology maintained its connection with objective abnormalities, but abandoned the mental disorders like schizophrenia, depression, and mania. Psychiatry became the specialty of the unknown. Psychotherapy and psychoanalysis relied on observing and interpreting human behaviour. There was no interest in the internal physiology of the brain.

In the past fifty years, the biological underpinnings of depression, anxiety, and other mental illness have been elucidated. Physical treatments such as electroconvulsant therapy (ECT) or biological treatments, such as antidepressant drugs, were found to be effective in depression. The genetic influences of diseases like schizophrenia and depression were appreciated. Studies of twins revealed that 30–60 percent of personality determinants were genetically inherited. Neuro-biological research revealed that specific chemical and electrical changes in the brain correlated with depressed mood.

Serotonin, already discussed as an important player in fibromyalgia, has been extensively studied in depression. Serotonin is a chemical found in plants and in many parts of our body and brain. It affects pain perception, as already discussed, in fibromyalgia. It enhances deep, restorative sleep. Serotonin controls the diameter of blood vessels and influences platelet aggregation, factors important in migraine headaches. Serotonin helps to regulate intestinal motility, a key factor in IBS. Serotonin is also involved in appetite, sexual interest, and cognition.

Serotonin is one of the most important neurotransmitters in mood disturbances. Reduced levels of serotonin or changes in serotonin receptor sites are found in depression. The efficacy of all antidepressants is based on increasing serotonin and other neurohormones. The tricyclic antidepressants and the selective serotonin reuptake inhibitors act by blocking the removal of serotonin at nerve synapses.

Sarah and I reviewed the similar physiological changes in depression and fibromyalgia. Brain-blood imaging using MRI, SPECT, and PET scans have demonstrated physiological abnormalities in mood disturbances similar to those in fibromyalgia and CFS. Depressed patients have orthostatic hypotension (fall in blood pressure) and exaggerated heart rate variability similar to that noted in fibromyalgia and CFS. This autonomic nervous system dysregulation may be important in the higher mortality rates seen when depressed heart attack patients are compared with non-depressed heart attack patients.

Low levels of serotonin have been demonstrated in the central nervous system in fibromyalgia and in depressed patients. A single dose of sertraline (Lustral) resulted in enhanced pain tolerance and increased cerebral blood flow in fibromyalgia patients. The blunted response of the hypothalamic-pituitary-adrenal stress axis in some fibromyalgia patients is similar to that found in melancholic depression.

The genetic predisposition for both illnesses, fibromyalgia and depression, could be linked to neurohormones like serotonin. Serotonin receptor genes are being studied in families with these disorders. Certain families may have genetic factors that make them predisposed to a spectrum of serotonin-deficiency illnesses, including fibromyalgia, depression, CFS, IBS, and migraine.

Gradually, Sarah accepted that her physical and emotional

symptoms were tied together. They shared biological alterations. Sarah made up a little poem:

> It's so good to find out
> It's not all in my head.
> Rather, my neurotransmitters
> Are acting wacky instead.

People with fibromyalgia and CFS are reluctant to acknowledge that depression is an important component of their illness. When they do, it is considered a normal reaction to their medical condition. Sarah and Virginia both declared: *I am depressed because of the fibromyalgia. Who wouldn't be?* This reactive depression is often contrasted to an endogenous depression, one thought to be biological. We now know that such a division is arbitrary. There is no such thing as a biological depression, best treated with medicine, and a psychological depression, best treated with psychotherapy. All depression is both biologically and environmentally determined.

Not recognizing and treating depression associated with fibromyalgia, CFS, and chronic pain may be fatal. On Friday, 17 August, 1996, three reporters from Boston television stations and newspapers phoned me in my office, frantically seeking my opinion about the latest suicide assisted by Dr. Jack Kevorkian. I knew nothing about it, so they told me that a Massachusetts woman who had fibromyalgia and CFS had committed suicide in Michigan with the help of Kevorkian.

Knowing nothing about the case, I was reluctant to make any comments. However, I did state that 'it's distressing to hear that someone took this desperate action.' I further told the reporter that I had treated patients, like Sarah, who told me that they had thought of killing themselves. Two patients with fibromyalgia had actually committed suicide years after I had seen them. The reporters pressed me to use this in their story. I was reluctant, but agreed provided they mentioned that these two suicides were the only ones of the ten thousand patients with fibromyalgia that I had seen in the previous eighteen years. I wanted to be certain that the public knew just how rare suicide was in these illnesses. But I also know personally and professionally the torment of chronic pain and medical uncertainty, and that such despair and depression can indeed drive someone to consider suicide.

Fibromyalgia, CFS, and chronic pain are never fatal in themselves, but an associated depression can be fatal. The Kevorkian-assisted suicide of a fibromyalgia/CFS patient was shocking. It is especially tragic in illnesses that aren't terminal and are treatable. But I have a healthy respect for the ravages of depression. Untreated major depression is a time bomb ready to explode.

It comes as no surprise that depression is a very important prognostic outcome factor in fibromyalgia. Pre-existing mood disturbances such as major depression or anxiety disorder are the single most important factor in determining whether an individual with musculoskeletal pain will subsequently be diagnosed to have fibromyalgia and will require treatment in a specialty clinic. Concurrent mood disturbances are one of the most important factors to predict how a fibromyalgia patient will respond to any form of treatment.

Sarah had many concerns about staying on antidepressant medication. Most of my patients voice the same feelings. There is an unhealthy fear about these drugs. They are no more likely to cause side effects than any other biologically active agent. I told Sarah that taking medications for depression and anxiety is no different than taking insulin for diabetes, or thyroid hormone for the treatment of hypothyroidism. Statistics reveal that 50 percent of patients with depression do not take their prescribed drug treatment. In part, this non-compliance is due to unpleasant drug effects, but mainly it reflects lack of understanding about these drugs. People worry that antidepressants blunt their real emotions or change their personality. Sarah commented: *I want to feel my emotions, be they happy or sad. I need to be able to grieve.* Antidepressant medications rarely block 'normal' emotional responses. They do filter out abnormal and excessive emotions, and so can relieve immense suffering.

Sarah has been taking SSRIs, the selective serotonin inhibitors. These include fluoxetine (Prozac), sertraline (Lustral), paroxetine (Seroxat), and citalopram (Lipramil). The older tricyclics like amitriptyline and the newer SSRIs are equally effective, but the SSRIs tend to have fewer side effects. They have less drowsiness, dryness, or cardiac problems than the tricyclics. SSRIs may cause a loss of libido. People who do not respond to these can often benefit from monoamine oxidase inhibitors (MAOs), but these medications impose various dietary restrictions. Lithium is the drug most often prescribed in bipolar depression. Certain anti-convulsants, such as gabepentin (Neurontin), carbamazepine (Tegretol), and sodium valproate (Epilim), may help to stabilize mood and may diminish pain.

As we better understand the genetic and biological aspects of depression and fibromyalgia, we can't lose sight of their psycho-social influences. A purely biochemical explanation of depression ignores the profound effect of our surroundings on our mind and body. If personal problems pile up, medications are not sufficient therapy. We need to examine our problems. We need to find solutions with the help of doctors, counsellors, friends, and family.

Even mental health experts dichotomize their therapies. Some psychiatrists now only prescribe medicine, with little counselling. People are in and out in ten minutes. Other mental health-care professionals don't believe in using antidepressants. They contend that psychotherapy and self-awareness are the real cures. To them, taking a pill is only a temporary solution. Family doctors and their patients may be caught in the middle.

The artificial gap between medical and psychiatric illnesses is narrowing. The most common illnesses like fibromyalgia, CFS, and IBS, do not fit snugly into either box.

Sarah responded best to a combination of biological (drugs) and psychological (counselling) therapy. I screen all of my fibromyalgia patients for mood disturbances. I often consult with a psychiatrist (see Table on Treatment, page 134). Counselling is directed at current symptom relief and based on cognitive behavioural changes. Sarah learned better coping mechanisms. Over time, she recognized the sense of peace that the medications and counselling provided. During her visit last year, she said: *I finally recognize the importance of taking my medicines. Knowing that depression is a chemical disturbance and what it has done to me makes it easier to accept the daily ritual of my drugs. All my life I felt strong, with a need to be fiercely independent. Now I accept my own frailties and appreciate the help of my doctors and my family. My mind and life are finally coming into balance.*

FICTION

- Fibromyalgia is simply a physical expression of depression and anxiety.

- Depression in fibromyalgia is a normal reaction to chronic illness.

- Depression is biological in some people and psychological in others.

- All fibromyalgia patients should be treated with antidepressants.

FACTS

- Fibromyalgia is not a psychiatric illness. Of patients with fibromyalgia, 30 percent are currently depressed and 70 percent have been depressed in their lives.

- Many of the pain complaints and sleep and cognitive disturbances in depression are similar to those in fibromyalgia.

- Depression is common in any chronic illness. It increases the risk of developing fibromyalgia. It adversely affects the outcome and must always be treated.

- There is a genetic predisposition to depression and to fibromyalgia. These two illnesses may be biologically linked.

- Counselling and supportive therapy is just as important as drug treatment in the outcome of people with depression and fibromyalgia.

10

How Does Stress Affect Me?

DAVID came to see me last year. He had been diagnosed with fibromyalgia by a rheumatologist at an army medical centre in 1996. I reviewed his files. David complained of persistent body aches, exhaustion, insomnia, and difficulty concentrating. These symptoms began soon after he had served in the Gulf War.

David walked into my office with a halting gait. Tall, lean, and wearing jeans, a motorcycle jacket, and army boots, he looked capable of riding his motorcycle across the country. Yet his facial expression implied otherwise as he grimaced with each step. David grew up in rural Vermont, one of seven children. He joined the army at the age of eighteen in 1983, and was medically discharged in 1991. He described what had happened to him:

I was never sick in my life before returning from the Gulf War. During the first few months back home I was tired, but figured that was normal. Then, little by little, I started feeling downright exhausted and began having bad muscle and joint pains. I got a rash on my hands and face. In the past year, I've fallen apart. My eyes are dry and get blood red and painful. My chest hurts all the time. I have trouble breathing. My bowels get all bound up and I feel sick a lot. My balance is off and I'm dizzy. Sometimes I feel hypoglycaemic and shake like a leaf unless I eat. My sleep is terrible, and when I do sleep, I have nightmares. The doctors at the army hospital ran a series of tests and said everything was okay. But I just felt worse and worse.

Some of my army mates had the same complaints. Then reports on TV and the news about Gulf War syndrome started. Some vets were coming down with bleeding gums, paralysis, and even cancer. I went back to the army hospital and the doctors said my symptoms had nothing to do with my time in the Gulf. Eventually, I was sent to a specialist who was studying Gulf War syndrome. After a week of every imaginable test he told me that I had fibromyalgia, whatever that is.

David's symptoms were typical of veteran soldiers (vets) diagnosed with Gulf War syndrome: unexplained exhaustion, cognitive disturbances, generalized body pain, headaches, diarrhoea, dizziness, sleep, and mood problems. These symptoms are indistinguishable from those of fibromyalgia and CFS. When I examined David, he had the characteristic tender points of fibromyalgia. The rest of his physical and neurological examination was normal. I agreed with the rheumatologist who diagnosed fibromyalgia. Exactly why this developed shortly after David returned from the Gulf War was unclear.

Approximately 10 percent of the seven hundred thousand U.S. troops who were in the Gulf have reported symptoms like David's. This number of sixty thousand sick vets sounds excessive. However, this is the exact number of people in the population at large with chronic pain and exhaustion. The prevalence of fibromyalgia, IBS, headaches, and mood disturbances in the population as a whole is approximately 10 percent.

This does not exclude the very real possibility that some Gulf War vets may have experienced a unique, new disease. Gulf War vets have developed illnesses such as cancer or arthritis, but at rates no greater than would be expected in the general population.

Subsequent comprehensive scientific studies from 1995 to the present found that Gulf War vets were not dying or being hospitalized at rates greater than vets who did not serve in the Gulf. Recently, studies suggest that there may be more cases of amyotrophic lateral sclerosis (Lou Gehrig's disease) in Gulf War vets, but this accounts for symptoms in only a handful of vets.

To date, $115 million has been spent on 120 research studies regarding Gulf War syndrome. Each study concluded that there is no single cause of the vets' symptoms. Possible causative factors of the Gulf War symptoms that have been evaluated include tropical infectious diseases, the many vaccinations and medications that the vets had received, biological weapons, depleted uranium, and pesticides. No toxic agent has been linked to the vets' symptoms.

David felt strongly that his symptoms were caused by a toxic substance that he had been exposed to in the Gulf. David suspected that the CIA and United States military lied about what happened in the Gulf. He said: *It's all part of their cover-up so that we don't sue them,* and quoted from Patrick Eddington's 1997 book *Gassed in the Gulf: The Inside Story of the Pentagon-CIA Cover-Up of Gulf War Syndrome.* Eddington, an analyst in the Directorate of Intelligence of the CIA, declared that secret documents, 'prove that tens of thousands of American troops had been exposed to deadly chemical agents . . . these chemicals are at least partly responsible for the chronic illnesses suffered by over one hundred thousand Desert Storm veterans . . . and for the birth defects among so many of their postwar children.'

Despite such books and media accusations, no unique new diseases have cropped up in Gulf War vets. Most vets were suffering from idiopathic chronic muscle and joint pain, profound fatigue, sleep disturbances, bowel disturbances, depression, headaches, and memory problems. Like David, many had fibromyalgia. In fact, the only illness found to be greater in Gulf War vets than in control subjects was fibromyalgia, present in one-third of ill vets examined by a rheumatologist.

I told David that the intense physical and emotional stress of the Gulf War may have triggered his illness. He was not satisfied with this explanation. No answers were coming from the military, from the Department of Defense, or from outside scientists. This only increased David's anger and fear. Then doctors told him that this was all psychological and not a physical reaction. None of us wants to hear that, particularly vets who served their country and put their lives on the line. As David said: *Any talk of stress means they are trying to tell me I'm nuts. That stress argument is the government's way to defuse the situation. I have never been depressed in my life. I had been in the military for years and never panicked. This is a disease that has never been seen before and we all got it in the same place. How could it be psychological if so many other vets have the same disease?*

David's response was identical to that of one of the Gulf War vets interviewed by Jeff Wheelwright in his book *The Irritable Heart:* 'John would never accept that his mind could be so powerful as to cause tremors and pain throughout his body. To him, as to most people, physical symptoms driven by the mind indicated a failure of character, a defective personality, rather than a genuine illness.'

David's symptoms were not unique. They were the same complaints that I saw daily in my patients with fibromyalgia and CFS. These same symptoms also have been reported by veterans of the American Civil War, the two world wars, and the Vietnam War. Heart damage was suspected as a cause of exhaustion in vets after the Civil War and World War I. The terms 'irritable heart' and 'Da Costa syndrome' were used, but no evidence for heart disease was found. In World Wars I and II, some vets with chronic fatigue, headaches, and muscle pain were diagnosed with Effort syndrome or 'neurocirculatory asthenia' (terms very similar to the diagnosis of neurasthenia in chronic fatigue sufferers). Dr. Paul Wood, a famous cardiologist, found no evidence for organic disease and suggested that psychological factors were involved.

Then, during World War II and the Vietnam War, the prevailing medical opinion shifted to psychological causes of combat-induced illness. 'Battle fatigue' was coined for acute, combat stress in World War II and 'posttraumatic stress disorder' was diagnosed in many veterans of the Korean and Vietnam Wars. Exposure to Agent Orange, a herbicide, was explored as a potential cause of the Vietnam symptoms. But this was a factor in a very small number of Vietnam veterans who became ill. The debate regarding physical or psychological causes of vets' illnesses has carried over to the current controversy about the Gulf War syndrome.

David was sick and he was hurting. He had been healthy before serving in the Gulf and came back ill. Anyone would jump to the conclusion that a Gulf germ or exposure to chemicals had made him sick. However, science has not backed such assumptions. Dr. Simon Wessely stated in Jane Brody's 16 March, 1999 *New York Times* report: 'Going to the Persian Gulf definitely affected the health of servicemen. We showed very considerable health effects. But that doesn't mean the disease they contracted is unique to science. They have legitimate health problems, but there is no single illness or single cause.'

Dr. Steven Joseph, then Assistant Secretary of Defense, cautioned: 'When the Presidential Advisory Committee brought out the issue of psychological stress in this whole equation, they were shouted down. Why is it so difficult to accept the message that when you put young Americans, or anyone, in a situation that is uncomfortable, dangerous, and uncertain, that a number of those people come back from that situation with a combination of physical symptoms and psychological symptoms. In a way I think that the greatest tragedy of the whole Gulf War illness issues is that we really had a chance . . . to understand and speak honestly and prepare ourselves for the mind–body combination of symptoms that always follows an armed conflict.'

David grudgingly listened to my comments about the consequences of severe stress. Humans and all living creatures survive by maintaining a complex, ever-changing equilibrium. Stress, which is best defined as a state of disharmony, threatens that homeostasis. Stressors can be metabolic (e.g., low blood sugar), physical (e.g., surgery and anaesthesia), or emotional (e.g., a tragic event). War triggers all three.

Medical science has focused on the psychological effects from stress. Stress had initially been examined within a psychosomatic framework. This implied that stress was a product of cognition and could be controlled by our free will. Psychiatrists gained prestige and cornered the market for stress treatment when they successfully used psychotherapy to treat soldiers with battle fatigue in World War II.

In the 1920s Walter Cannon, a Harvard neurologist, and his pupil Hans Selye, demonstrated that specific physical responses result from stress. In acute, self-limited stress, we become more alert, our hearts beat faster, our breathing becomes deeper. Our immunological and inflammatory responses are dampened. These changes help to protect us from acute injuries or infections. This is called 'the fight or flight reaction.'

When stress is chronic, such as during a prolonged illness, a maladaptive physiological and psychological response may develop. Chronic stress suppresses the appetite, causes loss of libido, inadequate body temperature regulation, exhaustion, disturbed sleep, and heightened pain perception. The arousal and alertness of acute stress is replaced by anxiety, hypervigilance, and chronic insomnia during chronic stress. The intense focus of our thoughts in acute stress gives way to obsessive thoughts, memory loss, and melancholia during chronic stress.

The stress response is controlled by the two competing branches of the autonomic nervous system. The sympathetic branch speeds things up, and the parasympathetic branch slows things down. Every gland, hormone, and neurotransmitter that I have mentioned is involved in regulating our stress response. The hypothalamus is the control switch. The hypothalamus is a gland embedded in the limbic system of our brain. The limbic system, often called the 'seat of our emotions,' relays messages to the endocrine and immune systems as well as to the autonomic nervous system. Neurohormones, such as ACTH, CRH, cortisol, adrenaline, noradrenaline, serotonin, cytokines, and endogenous opioids, relay the messages. There is constant cross-talk between the immune system and the central nervous system. Synchronized feedback coordinates these physiological responses to stress.

During chronic and persistent stress we feel constant muscle tension. Our heart rate is elevated. Our insides feel shaky. Our stomachs are upset – we experience 'butterflies' in our stomachs. We have sweaty palms. We are irritable.

Chronic stress increases our susceptibility to infection and prolongs recovery time. People who contracted the Asian flu during the epidemic of 1957 were three times more likely to have pre-existing anxiety and depression than those who did not get sick. Exposure to a common virus results in infection more often in people with high levels of pre-existing stress compared with those with lower stress levels. People taking care of relatives with Alzheimer's disease have a profoundly lowered immune response. Women who experience high levels of marital stress have a three-fold higher incidence of heart attacks than women without such stress.

Hans Selye observed: 'Overwhelming stress can break down the body's protective mechanisms. It is for this reason that so many maladies tend to be rampant during wars and famines. If a microbe is in or around us all the time and yet causes no disease until we are exposed to stress, what is the cause of illness, the microbe or the stress? I think both are – and equally so.'

Stress has a major impact on heart disease and heart attacks. It was always known that the so-called Type-A personality was more prone to develop heart attacks. There have been numerous studies demonstrating that strong emotions can trigger heart attacks. Emotional or physical stress causes a surge of adrenaline and noradrenaline with resultant blood pressure and heart rate elevations. Anger, grief, and fear are as important as the known physical triggers such as an elevated cholesterol.

David and I set about changing his reaction to stress. We

reviewed studies that have demonstrated the powerful effects of stress reduction. Stress reduction lowers blood pressure and pulse. How we respond to stress is not fixed. It is also possible to change our immune response. An experimental autoimmune disease in mice, very similar to systemic lupus erythematosus (lupus) in humans, was used to document the powerful influence of the mind on immune disease. Mice with lupus were treated with Cytoxan, an immunosuppressive medication that controlled the lupus. They then learned to associate each dose of the drug with drinking a sweet fluid. Eventually, just the drink alone produced the same, powerful, immune beneficial effects on the animals' lupus as did the Cytoxan.

This was one of the first studies to convince scientists that the brain and the nervous system can have a direct influence on the immune system. Such studies have led to the development of the exciting field of psycho-neuroimmunology. It is now thought that we can each potentially learn ways to modify our own stress response and, through that, our immune response. When capsaicin, the active ingredient in hot chilli peppers, is applied to the skin of a person with fibromyalgia, the inflammatory reaction is greater than in normal individuals. This exaggerated immune response was blunted when the fibromyalgia patients learned stress-reduction techniques. Rather than automatically reacting to stress in a negative fashion, we can learn techniques to dampen its adverse physiological effects.

Personally, I had never paid much attention to stress until my recurrent illnesses a few years ago. In retrospect, many of my bouts of fatigue followed major stress. I had a severe, flu-like illness that persisted for three months thirty years ago. This hit me in the middle of my training as a junior doctor, a year of forced sleep deprivation and unrealistic physical and intellectual demands. My chronic headaches and insomnia that began ten years ago developed during a time of stress triggered by a major career change. The bout of depression came on the heels of brain surgery.

It was at that time that I began meditation and yoga techniques, which are designed to relax the brain and the body. Relaxation decreases activity in the sympathetic nervous system, and the 'fight or flight' response. I had witnessed the powerful effects of stress reduction during a programme for patients with fibromyalgia and arthritis at a popular health spa in Tucson, Arizona. A daily programme of exercise and relaxation techniques, including yoga, meditation, and tai-chi, along with educational sessions, were provided for the patients. Measures of stress reactivity and immune function were taken before and after the programme. Following the intervention, there were significant improvements in baseline stress reactions as well as in immune function. Because I was exercising on a regular basis, I decided to add relaxation techniques to my daily schedule.

Relaxation techniques include biofeedback, hypnosis, meditation, yoga, prayer, tai-chi, chi-gong, and deep breathing with imagery or repetitive exercise. These techniques require the person to concentrate on repetitive words, sounds, prayer, or body sensations, and to clear the mind of intruding thoughts. Anything that initiates the relaxation response can be useful. The relaxation response results in lowered heart rate, decreased blood pressure, and a diminished response to the typical stress hormones. Following biofeedback or meditation there is also a shift in brain wave activity towards less arousal and greater calm.

David began to understand the negative impact of chronic stress on his health. He commented, *I began to think that I would never get better. Why was this happening to me? It just wasn't fair. I was angry all the time. Now I have more of a handle on life in general. I have learned to put things in perspective.*

We will always have stress. Hans Selye said 'stress is life and life is stress.' Our response to stress is in part inherited and in part acquired. Children of Holocaust survivors were found to have exaggerated stress responses despite not going through any of the horrors of their parents. But how we react to stress can be modified. Stress doesn't necessarily cause disease, but contributes significantly to its impact on each of us. Finding healthier ways to deal with our stress will go a long way to taking charge of our symptoms rather than allowing them to take hold of us.

FICTION

- Gulf War syndrome is a unique new disease.

- Some of us just can't handle stress.

- Stress is a purely psychological reaction.

FACTS

- Every war has been followed by vets becoming ill with symptoms that are typical of fibromyalgia.

- Stress causes a cascade of physical and psychological responses, some beneficial, some harmful.

- Chronic stress causes hyperarousal and immune system dysfunction.

- Stress responses can be modified by relaxation techniques and cognitive behavioural therapy.

11

What Medications Should I Take?

JONATHAN'S primary symptom was pain. Denise complained most bitterly of feeling exhausted all of the time. Patty was tormented as much by insomnia as by pain and fatigue. The treatment of fibromyalgia requires treating each of its major symptoms. One medication may work better for pain whereas another may work only for the sleep disturbances.

The medical treatment for fibromyalgia must be highly individualized (see Table on Treatment, page 134). Most of the time, I prescribe medications for the relief of pain, to improve energy, and to improve sleep. Some medications are capable of doing all three.

During most of the past fifty years, the treatment of pain has been relegated to second-class status in medicine. Other than anaesthetists treating perioperative pain or oncologists easing the pain associated with cancer, specific pain management has been an ignoble practice. Physicians have been trained to search for the cause of pain and eradicate it. When no cause of chronic pain is found, its treatment has been frustrating and at times quite futile. Chronic pain patients have been misunderstood, pitied, or rejected.

Accepting and treating chronic pain as an entity in itself is gaining more momentum. Hospitals now mandate that every patient's pain levels are recorded daily with other vital signs, such as temperature, blood pressure, and heart rate. Most hospitals in the United States have pain management teams. Nevertheless, a tiny fraction of research dollars are spent on understanding and treating pain. Basic mechanisms of pain are rarely taught in medical schools.

The three major classes of pain relievers (analgesics) are the nonsteroidal anti-inflammatory agents (known as NSAIDs), the opioid analgesics, and anaesthetics.

ANTI-INFLAMMATORY ANALGESICS
The anti-inflammatory analgesics, such as the NSAIDs, relieve pain and also chemically block the inflammation process. Corticosteroids, such as prednisone, are the most powerful anti-inflammatory drugs. Anti-inflammatory medications are best used for the pain of diseases like rheumatoid arthritis that involve inflammation of joints, muscles, or other tissues. Fibromyalgia, CFS, and chronic headaches are rarely associated with inflammation, so steroids and NSAIDs are of limited use. Steroids have considerable toxicity and little efficacy as pain relievers, but NSAIDs can be analgesic even at low doses. Low doses of NSAIDs like ibuprofen or naproxen can 'take the edge off pain' and are quite safe, although, with long-term use, gastrointestinal or kidney problems may occur. Paracetamol has no major risk of ulcers or bleeding and may be just as helpful to decrease pain. Unfortunately, none of the NSAIDs or even steroids decreased Jon's pain.

Jonathan also participated in clinical trials with new anti-inflammatory medications called Cox 2 inhibitors. These drugs selectively block the second cyclo-oxygenase enzyme in contrast to all of the prior anti-inflammatory medications, which also block the first enzyme. Both of these enzymes are important in pain and in tissue inflammation. Selectively blocking Cox 2 results in less gastrointestinal bleeding, ulcers, or gastritis. These medications are also long acting, providing twenty-four-hour analgesia with a single dose, which is an advantage in the treatment of chronic pain.

If anti-inflammatory medications have any efficacy in fibromyalgia, it is related to their central nervous system analgesic effects. They also may be useful when fibromyalgia patients have co-existing arthritis or bursitis. The other analgesic that Jonathan tried with little success was tramadol (Zydol). Tramadol has a central nervous system analgesic effect as an opioid agonist (stimulus) and also it inhibits serotonin and noradrenaline reuptake. It may help to reduce pain, but usually needs to be taken at high doses three times each day.

OPIOID ANALGESICS

During the four years before I began treating Jon, he had been taking oxycodone and other opioid analgesics. The use of opium for pain relief can be traced back to the Egyptians in 1550 B.C. Opium is extracted from poppy seed pods and contains many pain relieving compounds, including those found in morphine, codeine, and drugs such as oxycodone. Opioids reduce pain by their effect on specific receptors in the brain and spinal cord.

The most commonly prescribed opioids in the United States include morphine, codeine, oxycodone, meperidine, methadone, and propxyphene. They can be administered by injection, intravenously, orally, under the tongue, or through skin absorption, as with the fentanyl (Durogesic) patch. New opioids that have less toxicity are in the pipeline. Opioid analgesics act on both the sensory as well as emotional components of pain. Most opioids are compared in potency with morphine, a relatively pure opioid agonist. Hydrocodone and morphine have a relatively short half-life. Oxycodone (OxyContin) and transdermal fentanyl have a twelve to seventy-two hour effect.

Opioids are the most effective pain relievers, but fear of addiction limits their use. Jon had been cautioned repeatedly about his 'dependency' on oxycodone. Much of the fear of addiction is greatly exaggerated in patients with chronic pain. True addiction is primarily limited to people with a history of drug, alcohol, or other substance abuse. Drug tolerance, wherein escalating amounts of the drug are necessary to achieve the same response, does develop in some people. Anyone on opioids is prone to drug withdrawal symptoms, but withdrawal is manageable if doses are slowly tapered before they are discontinued. Many drugs that affect pain, sleep, mood, or cognition may cause unpleasant or even dangerous reactions if they are abruptly discontinued.

Jon never took more opioids than prescribed. In fact, he usually tried to skip doses so, as he said, '*I would not become dependent on narcotics.*' Paradoxically, taking opioids in this fashion is more likely to create psychological dependency. Patients and doctors need to understand that opioids should not be used as needed. Rather, they should be dosed continuously so their analgesic effect does not peak and fall. It is the erratic use of opioids that creates more problems, especially drug withdrawal. Jon complained of more pain and became quite anxious whenever he stopped taking oxycodone. He angrily responded, *My doctors said that each operation would take care of the pain. But I just got worse. Once the surgeons couldn't help, they got tired of seeing me. They sent me to another doctor who did more X-rays and MRIs. More than one doctor told me that I was becoming a druggie. I hated taking oxycodone all the time, but it was the only way I could get through the day. Now you want to take away the only thing that keeps me going. I don't trust anyone anymore.*

I consulted with my colleagues in our pain management programme and I switched Jon from oxycodone to Durogesic (fentanyl patch), administered every three days. Jon subsequently had much less breakthrough pain. Longer-acting analgesics have been more effective with less need for drug escalation than short-acting drugs, like Percocet. Percocet, a combination of paracetamol and the opioid, oxycodone, only works for three or four hours. Although widely used in the United States, it is not available in

Britain. I also added dextromethorphan, the 'DM' of Robitussin-DM, which further decreased his pain. Dextromethorphan blocks chemical receptors called NMDA, which are important in initiating central sensitization.

ANAESTHETICS AND OTHER ANALGESICS

It is hard to conceive of the world of medicine without anaesthesia. However, the first use of anaesthesia during surgery was in 1846. Although anaesthesia has revolutionized pain control during surgery, it has been of limited use for the treatment of chronic pain. Patients with fibromyalgia and myofascial pain do often receive pain relief when anaesthetics such as lidocaine are injected in tender points or trigger points.

Jonathan's pain improved with trigger point injections. An anaesthetic (lidocaine) was injected into areas of the muscle that were especially taut and tender. These injections work best when followed by muscle stretching and movement, what Dr. Janet Travell calls myofascial release. Trigger point injections are very safe and can relieve local muscle spasm and pain, although the improvement usually only lasts for days. Anaesthetics, like lidocaine, given intravenously or topically, can also be used to treat chronic pain, but unpleasant side effects and their very short action have limited their value.

I then began Jon on Neurontin (gabepentin) as well as amitriptyline at bedtime. Anticonvulsants, such as Neurontin, interfere with neuronal activity that is important in pain transmission. Tricyclic antidepressants such as amitriptyline and imipramine have various analgesic actions, including suppressing nerve cell discharge and inhibiting serotonin and noradrenaline reuptake. The addition of these two medications allowed me to gradually wean Jon off opioids during the next year.

OTHER MEDICATIONS

Denise was much more affected by exhaustion. After she had tried megavitamins, antibiotics, antiviral agents, and numerous intravenous infusions, she reluctantly agreed to try sertraline (Lustral). I began her on 25 mg of sertraline (Lustral) in the morning, an extremely low dose, and gradually increased it to 100 mg every morning. Denise did not meet criteria for major depression. The doses of antidepressants that have been used to improve energy are typically lower than the doses used for the treatment of depression. Certain antidepressants, especially the SSRIs such as sertraline, fluoxetine, and paroxetine may be more helpful in restoring energy than other antidepressants.

Patty's sleep disturbances triggered her exhaustion and her pain. Most patients with fibromyalgia and CFS have disturbances in deep, stage 4 sleep. Primary sleep disorders such as sleep apnea or restless leg syndrome are not uncommon. If there is any concern about such sleep disorders, the patient should be referred to a sleep clinic and have an overnight sleep study.

After just one night of taking 20 mg of amitriptyline, a tricyclic antidepressant, Patty felt better than she had in months. Her sleep disturbances were so overwhelming that as soon as she got better, and deeper, sleep she improved. During the past twenty years, she has taken a small amount of amitriptyline, usually between 20 to 30 mg at night, to maintain an adequate and refreshing night of sleep. Antidepressant drugs such as amitriptyline and cyclobenzaprine are more effective than placebo and more effective than NSAIDs for pain relief as well as overall well-being in fibromyalgia. They have been used in low doses and usually at night. We start people on amitriptyline 10 mg one or two hours before bedtime and typically go no higher than 30 mg.

Patty has tried other medications because of the nuisance side effects, such as constipation, with tricyclic antidepressants. But nothing has been as effective. The tricyclic compounds have an analgesic effect that is different from their antidepressant action. The sleep promoting and analgesic effects fortunately kick in at lower doses than their antidepressant effects. Therefore, adverse side effects tend to be manageable, although reactions such as dry mouth, fluid retention, weight gain, tachycardia and sedation can be intolerable for some people. Patty puts up with the dryness, constipation, and increased appetite these medications cause. The trade-off to get deep, refreshing sleep and to have less muscle pain has been worth it for her.

Other antidepressants, such as venlafaxine (Effexor) and, trazodone (Molipaxin) can be useful. At night, clonazepam (Rivotril), 0.5 to 1 mg, or lorazepam (Ativan), 0.5 to 1 mg, have been very helpful in treating sleep disturbances. These benzodiazepines or L-Dopa/carbidopa (Sinemet) are the best drugs to treat restless leg syndrome, a periodic leg movement disorder that interrupts sleep in about 5 percent of the population. In addition to easing anxiety and insomnia, benzodiazepines may help decrease pain because of direct analgesic action on the brain. As with opioids, there are concerns about addiction with these benzodiazepine medications. However, if these drugs are kept at low doses, addiction does not occur. Zolpidem (Stilnoct) is helpful in treating fibromyalgia sleep disturbances, although it does not lessen muscle pain. Melatonin is often used to help sleep and helps short-term problems such as jet lag. Our research demonstrated that fibromyalgia patients do not have a deficiency in melatonin. Melatonin was not effective in the treatment of fibromyalgia symptoms in a randomized clinical trial. Modafinil (Provigil), a new wakefulness-promoting drug, may help the fatigue in some patients.

Side effects of these drugs can be minimized and their efficacy heightened with a combination of medications, each given at a low dose. A patient might take a low, morning dose of one of the newer SSRIs, such as 10 mg of fluoxetine or 50 mg of sertraline (Lustral), combined with a low night time dose of tricyclic antidepressant, such as 10–25 mg of amitriptyline. Since the tricyclic medications and the SSRIs have different physiological effects on neurohormones such as serotonin and noradrenaline, combining different classes of drugs is logical.

Other common symptoms that occur in fibromyalgia may require different medications. Among people with fibromyalgia, one-third are depressed and need adequate antidepressant medications in therapeutic doses. The low doses of antidepressant or anxiolytic agents that I use to treat pain and the sleep disturbances would not suffice. Migraine headaches might respond best to one of the more specific medications such as the triptans. IBS is often treated with antispasmodics or one of the new 5-HT$_3$ antagonists. Irritable bladder syndrome has been treated with oxybutynin.

A number of over-the-counter medicinal products have been recommended to treat fibromyalgia. Although I will deal with this in greater detail in the next chapter, some fall under the category of medications. For example, magnesium and malic acid have been claimed to help diminish muscle pain in fibromyalgia. There is only one study on this combination and it was disappointing. The most widely touted agent is guaifenesin, which is found in many cough expectorants.

A California-based endocrinologist hypothesized that fibromyalgia is caused by too much uric acid and inorganic phosphates in muscle. He postulates that guaifenesin will get rid of these and thereby restore muscle energy. However, muscle biopsies and techniques such as MRI spectroscopy have not demonstrated any metabolic abnormalities of muscle. The single, randomized clinical trial of guaifenesin in fibromyalgia found that it was no more effective than placebo. Unless new research studies reveal different results, I do not routinely recommend guaifenesin as a primary treatment for fibromyalgia patients.

Many of my fibromyalgia patients report that they can't take any medication. They describe allergies or sensitivities to numerous types of drug. It has also been stated in various books that people with fibromyalgia and CFS are more allergic or more sensitive to medications of all classes. This has not been scientifically validated. Fibromyalgia patients are hypersensitive to heat or cold, loud noises, and bright lights. They also exhibit sensitivity to medications. This does not mean that the medications are dangerous to them or will create true allergic or anaphylactic reactions. I always introduce medications very slowly and carefully at the lowest dose possible. We also discuss the fact that anxiety about taking medications will increase the stress response. Stress physiologically mimics an adverse drug reaction.

As scientists develop a greater understanding of the mind and body pathways involved in chronic illness, more targeted drugs will become available. Such medications will interact specifically with a tiny target – and only that target – in the central nervous system. This means that such drugs will be more effective and cause fewer side effects. Development of new serotonin receptor antagonists is an active research area. One of them, tropisetron, looks promising in initial studies conducted in Germany. New substance P and NMDA antagonists are also being tested.

When Jon returned to see me this past year, he was much more animated. Bonnie no longer did his talking. He moved more freely and was in much less pain. He was working part-time repairing cars and taking evening classes at a community college. We had been able to gradually reduce his pain medications and he was no longer depressed. Although never fully free of pain, Jon had achieved a much more active, more productive and happier life.

Jon's experience with chronic pain parallels that of most of my patients with chronic illness. For more than ten years, Jon's life centred around getting rid of his pain. Once he learned that he could get on with living despite the pain, his whole existence changed. If I ask any of my patients to choose either relief from pain or a return to a more normal life, they will generally pick the latter. But most of us can't comprehend how we could live happily and feel productive if we are still in pain. Jon is testament to the fact that we can.

Current medications for fibromyalgia are only modestly helpful. We can be very hopeful that treatment will improve in the near future. As we get closer to understanding the complex interactions of chemicals that control pain and energy, we can expect more targeted drugs. The current medications used in fibromyalgia work best in combinations and in conjunction with many nonmedicinal therapies. Nevertheless, the complexity of these illnesses makes it unlikely that a 'silver bullet' will be found.

FICTION

- Narcotics should never be used to treat chronic pain.

- Every fibromyalgia patient should be treated with antidepressants.

- Patients should never take anti-anxiety medications such as benzodiazepines.

- Medications don't work.

FACTS

- Analgesics are useful, but only palliative. Opioids are necessary in a small percent of people with fibromyalgia and should be prescribed by pain management experts.

- Treatment should be directed at the symptoms that are most troublesome. Some medications are better for pain, others for sleep, others for energy. Certain drugs, such as the tricyclic antidepressants, help all of these symptoms.

- Anti-anxiety medications, such as the benzodiazepines, and low doses of SSRIs are helpful in many fibromyalgia patients.

- There is no best medication for any single fibromyalgia patient.

- The best approach is to try different medications, doses, and combinations.

12

What Other Treatment Is Helpful?

MEDICATIONS are only one part of an effective therapeutic programme for people with fibromyalgia. Every person with fibromyalgia needs to be as active as possible. Pain and muscle spasm interfere with daily activities and with exercise. Eventually muscle weakness, atrophy, and deconditioning set in. There are many techniques that may help to reduce muscle pain, increase flexibility, and maintain cardiovascular fitness. Jonathan had failed to improve with months of physical therapy and chiropractic treatment. His first physiotherapist used passive techniques, such as massage and ultrasound. Jon told me that his muscles felt good during the massage or physical therapy. Once he got back home, his muscles tightened up and the pain intensified. Unfortunately, this is often the case. While regular massage can help lessen muscle spasm, it gets expensive if you go to a professional therapist. I often recommended that the spouse learns to perform a good massage.

Jonathan described his experience with a chiropractor: *I started going to the chiropractor after my last operation in 1990. At first, it helped me more than anything. However, each time it seemed*

like cracking my back worked for shorter and shorter periods of
time. He then said that I had to come for more manipulations.
Several vertebrae in my back were out of place. Eventually I was
going to the chiropractor twice a week. This went on for two and
a half years until I couldn't afford it.

Chiropractic is the largest form of alternative medical practice
in the United States, although it has become mainstream with the
public. Chiropractors are licensed in all fifty states and one out of
three Americans with lower back pain has been treated by a chiropractor. Patients with low back pain consult a chiropractor more
often than orthopaedic surgeons or rheumatologists. There are
currently fifty thousand chiropractors in the United States and
that number is expected to double in ten years. In 1990 there were
160 million visits to chiropractors and 4 billion dollars were spent
on chiropractic care. Most insurance companies now reimburse
patients for treatment from a chiropractor.

Traditional medicine has rejected chiropractic care, although
this has started to change. Until recently, the American Medical
Association prohibited doctors from consulting with chiropractors. However, in 1994 the Agency for Health-care Policy in
Research declared that spinal manipulation can alleviate low
back pain. Much of the conflict with medical doctors results
from chiropractic's tenets that vertebrae commonly move out
of place or sublux. However, vertebrae never move substantially unless there is severe physical trauma. Chiropractors have
consistently maintained that vertebral subluxations and bone
displacements negatively affect mobility, posture and blood
flow, and often impinge upon spinal nerves causing 'vertebral
blockage.' Some chiropractors use manipulative therapy for
treating headaches, asthma, neurological diseases, and cancer.
This broad range of treatments has a lot to do with chiropractic's bad reputation with doctors. A recent report in children
with asthma found that chiropractic spinal manipulation provided no benefit.

There is evidence that chiropractic or osteopathic treatment can help a variety of musculoskeletal disorders, including fibromyalgia. Chiropractors and osteopaths have good hands. They understand how far to move muscles and joints. Their treatment often improves mobility. Many of my patients gain benefit from chiropractic and osteopathic care. While there have been very few randomized clinical trials using chiropractic or osteopathic manipulation, two recent studies demonstrated that chiropractic and physical therapy were equally effective in treating low back pain. However, they were each only marginally more effective than simply handing a brochure about low back pain to the patient.

Why is chiropractic effective if there is little scientific basis regarding its principles of treatment? Chiropractic comforts patients. Doctors can't tell fibromyalgia patients the cause of their symptoms. Chiropractors point to structural alterations as a clear-cut physical cause of people's pain. This explanation makes intuitive sense and also validates the patient's symptoms. Chiropractors and osteopaths touch patients much more than traditional physicians. Patients often have immediate personal feedback, such as hearing *pops* or *cracks* in their spines. This reinforces the notion that the manipulation is attacking the source of pain. Medical doctors can learn a lot from chiropractors in regard to the patient-doctor relationship.

Chiropractors, osteopaths, physiotherapists, and neuromuscular therapists address postural imbalances. Making people cognizant of how they sit, move, lift, and exercise reaps long-range benefits. Treatment should be of limited duration. No treatment for chronic pain should be indefinitely continued unless clear-cut improvement is seen.

The goal of physical therapy, whether treating fibromyalgia or chronic back pain, is to increase mobility, activity, and strength. This approach is in stark contrast to treatment of back pain during most of the past fifty years. Until recently, the theory was that the back was 'injured,' so it should be rested. Movement was to be avoided. Patients with back pain were often treated with prolonged bed rest, forced inactivity, back braces, or back traction. Doctors now recognize that the longer back movement is restricted, the more difficult it is to rehabilitate the back.

For people who grew up under the old approach, this new concept is sometimes difficult to grasp or accept. Jon's initial physical therapy was designed to strengthen his back and make him more active. It was started slowly. Each session included massage, ultrasound, and electrical stimulation. Strenuous workouts and sports medicine therapies are inappropriate for patients with fibromyalgia and CFS. There must be a very careful incremental rehabilitation when people have been suffering chronic pain and exhaustion for months or years. I asked Jon and Denise to consult with Dr. Joanne Borg-Stein, the rehabilitation specialist who is a key member of our treatment team.

TABLE 1
Treatment Principles in Fibromyalgia

ALWAYS:

Education session
* Group format
* Detailed didactic lecture
* Answer questions, concerns
* End with one-to-one advice

Advice on exercise and activity
* Cardiovascular exercise
* Stretching

USUALLY:

Medications
* Tricyclics (such as amitriptyline or dothiepin at night), SSRIs (such as fluoxetine)
* Analgesics (NSAIDs, paracetamol, tramadol)

OFTEN:

- Sleep medications
- Anti-anxiety medications
- Physical medicine, physical therapy referral
- Counselling, mental health professional referral

MORE PROBLEMATIC CASES

- Pain management clinic, rehabilitation programmes
- Cognitive behaviour, stress reduction programme

Many of my patients don't even know what a rehabilitation specialist or physiatrist is. They are physicians with a special interest in musculoskeletal and rehabilitation medicine. They are very adept at assessing anatomic and structural problems and performing techniques such as trigger point injections or acupuncture. They often direct departments of physical therapy.

Our rehabilitation specialist also used acupuncture, which gave Jon longer lasting relief. Acupuncture has been the most common medical procedure performed in China for the past two thousand years. The theory of acupuncture is based on the premise that patterns of energy, qi, flow through the body and acupuncture corrects imbalances in this flow. There are twelve primary qi channels or meridians. The acupuncture practitioner identifies the imbalance and selects among 360 acupuncture points distributed along these meridians. A long, thin needle is inserted manually at the acupuncture site although heat, pressure (acupressure), or electrical stimulation (electroacupuncture) have also become popular. Western medicine believes that acupuncture, as well as trigger point injections, decrease pain via actions of the central nervous system rather than the Eastern idea of energy imbalance. The bottom line is that acupuncture can work.

There are now seven studies of acupuncture in fibromyalgia, each reporting some benefit. Similar results have been noted in back pain and other musculoskeletal pain disorders. Acupuncture should be performed by someone who is well-trained;

there are about ten thousand licensed acupuncturists in the United States. Rehabilitation specialists are often trained in medical acupuncture.

Once Jon's pain lessened with trigger point injections and acupuncture, he began a progressive exercise programme. Gentle cardiovascular fitness exercise can greatly benefit most patients with chronic low back pain, fibromyalgia, and CFS. Often, patients who enjoyed exercise before becoming ill have stopped all kinds of activity because of their pain, fatigue, or fear that activity will make them worse. However, they usually find that the right approach to exercise makes them feel better. Although Jon had never previously participated in a regular exercise programme, he accepted the challenge to work with our physical rehabilitation and exercise group.

The goal of each of these physical techniques is to interrupt the vicious cycle of pain leading to muscle spasm, diminished blood supply, and more pain. Whether a treatment works locally, as with massage or trigger point injections, or systemically, such as with drugs, cardiovascular exercise, or biofeedback, is immaterial as long as it helps.

Cardiovascular exercise improves general fitness. It also can raise our spirits. A pain-relieving effect is noticeable with high levels of exercise. Intense exercise releases endorphins from the brain. Cardiovascular exercise also improves immune function and lessens susceptibility to infections. Even modest exercise reduces depression and increases energy. Studies suggest that the optimal time to exercise is in the late afternoon or early evening, but whatever fits into one's schedule will do.

A well-rounded exercise programme should include stretching and muscle strengthening. Stretching is especially important in people with fibromyalgia. Pain automatically forces muscles to tighten and go into spasm. This interferes with oxygen supply to the muscle. Tight muscles become shorter and their range of motion is decreased. Therefore muscles must be elongated. That is the goal of stretching. Patty and I stretch while we do simple yoga postures. Denise began yoga classes and found yoga very helpful.

Yoga means 'to bind together' or 'to concentrate.' Yoga symbolizes exercising the mind and body in harmony. The art of yoga, taught for over two thousand years in India, emphasizes the psychological aspects of healing. Specific postures and focused breathing or meditation calm the mind. I don't claim to be very flexible, and I have never been able to get my body into a lotus posture or do a headstand. But yoga does not necessarily require calisthenics or pretzel-like poses. I simply stretch in a slow and concentrated fashion using deep breathing. Many of my patients do yoga, tai-chi, chi-gong, or meditation. These exercises increase flexibility, strength, and body awareness. Most importantly, they focus our minds.

Learning to calm my mind and embrace stillness was very difficult for me. I hear the same thing from my patients. Denise told me that her mind was always racing. She was constantly worried about what she needed to do next or what she should have done in the past. Meditation and techniques such as yoga teach us to concentrate on the present moment. When I was able to attain that calmness, I felt very refreshed. This feeling of inner peace has much to do with the sudden popularity of meditation and yoga in Western culture.

Patty had always exercised regularly, but stopped exercising when she became ill. Jon had never done much exercise. They now know that exercise was very important in improving their health. It wasn't easy. Cardiovascular exercise was especially daunting to Denise. Her exhaustion worsened each time she took a walk. Some CFS support groups and Web sites claimed that vigorous exercise would damage her immune system. I reassured her that would not happen.

When you are exhausted, exercise is the last thing you feel like doing. Rest has been recommended for the treatment of CFS since it was called 'neurasthenia' in Victorian times. A paediatrician recently warned that CFS should be treated initially with 'total rest' and 'forcing a child to participate in normal, day-to-day activities will only make things worse. If the child has a rapid pulse or heartbeat, over-exertion can be very dangerous . . . so can exercising muscles before they're fully recovered, which, in extreme cases, can lead to paralysis.' This position is absurd and frightening to the child and her parents.

I explained to Denise that prolonged inactivity does have profound adverse physiological and psychological effects. The very symptoms of CFS, namely loss of stamina and strength, postural hypotension, and poor sleep are all made worse with bed rest. Furthermore, scientific studies in patients with fibromyalgia and CFS have noted beneficial effects with an exercise programme.

Denise joined one of our supervised exercise programmes. She reported:

I was so nervous when I began to exercise. I had been told that any exertion would aggravate my CFS. At first, even slow walking caused more aches and pains. But it felt like a 'good pain.' It was easier to tolerate than the pains from sitting around and doing nothing. These were what I called 'bad pains.' I learned to avoid certain activities and habits. Vacuuming killed my neck and shoulders. Since I hated to vacuum anyway, it wasn't a hardship to let someone else do it. My physiotherapist taught me water aerobics, which I now love. I also learned relaxation techniques. Sometimes, when I feel stressed and exhausted, I will stop what I'm doing and relax by listening to music. My energy is not the same as it was five years ago. But I've learned how to pace myself. My husband and children have also learned to respect my quiet time.

Any exercise programme should be carefully tailored to the patient's age and previous level of physical activity. A physiotherapist or personal trainer can plan the programme. Thirty minutes of moderately intense physical activities three or four days each week is recommended. Any exercise is better than none. Cardiovascular training, typically termed aerobic exercise, is most important. This can be walking, cycling, swimming, or similar activities.

A sufficient warm-up and cooldown is also important. Some form of strength training should gradually be introduced into an exercise programme. Options include: exercise balls, stretchable cords called Thera-Bands, or resistance machines and free weights.

Jon was taught to pay more attention to his posture and how he lifted heavy objects. Our rehabilitation specialist and co-workers watched Jon sit, get up, and walk. His back pain had produced tightness of his hip flexors. The limited flexibility of his lower back and legs made walking difficult and crooked. Jon had lost significant muscle strength in his lower abdomen and buttocks. He was taught postural realignment, hip flexion exercises, pelvic tilts, and modified sit-ups. He initially spent approximately thirty minutes three or four times a week doing flexibility exercises. Other body awareness and postural training techniques include the Alexander technique, Feldenkrais, and Pilates, which have increased in popularity in recent years.

Each time that I saw Jon in the office, we reviewed his response to medication and exercise. We talked about his cycle of chronic pain and inactivity. I explained to Jon that he needed to let go of the notion that his back pain was due to persistent tissue damage. Jon had anticipated that normal activities or any exercise would aggravate his pain. In his view, such activities needed to be avoided. He would tense up and become rigid as soon as he tried to do any physical activity, yet inactivity only worsened his chronic back pain.

Fibromyalgia patients often discontinue their exercise programmes and frequently tell me that their pain does not improve with exercise. However, the purpose of exercise is not to decrease pain, but rather to restore function and prevent further atrophy and injury. Occasionally there will be significant analgesic effect, probably through release of endorphins.

Counselling, via individual or group therapy, is often very helpful in fibromyalgia and related disorders (see Table on Treatment, page 134). Like Virginia, many patients with ill-defined illnesses suffer from unrealistic fears about a missed diagnosis or undiscovered diseases. This excess somatic concern is difficult to dismiss and is best handled with information and counselling. Unfortunately, family doctors and specialists often do not have sufficient time to explore these issues.

Mental health professionals are trained in counselling techniques. Some of my fibromyalgia patients have benefited from working with social workers, licensed clinical nurse specialists, occupational therapists, psychologists, or psychiatrists. Any patient with concurrent major depression or panic disorder, such as Sarah, should be referred to a psychiatrist who is skilled in psychopharmacology. Jane has joined a group programme for people with a history of physical or sexual trauma during childhood. Clearly, the treatment of fibromyalgia is dictated by the variety and severity of symptoms that the patient suffers.

FICTION

- Avoid too much activity; conserve your energy.

- Exercise should relieve pain; if it doesn't, don't exercise.

- Pain is caused by spinal subluxations.

- Push harder to get better results.

FACTS

- Pain and fatigue interfere with activity. Reduced activity increases pain.

- An ideal programme combines cardiovascular exercise, stretching, and strengthening. Exercise decreases spasm, increases blood flow, and restores function.

■ Physical therapy, chiropractic or osteopathic treatment, trigger point injections, and acupuncture are often helpful.

■ Yoga and meditation are cost-effective techniques that calm the mind and help physical and emotional flexibility.

■ Start slowly and get some professional guidance. It's okay to exercise up to normal pain and stiffness levels, but if your symptoms worsen, cut down the exercise.

13

What About Complementary and Natural Remedies?

MOST of my patients have tried alternative or complementary medical treatments. One survey estimated that 91 percent of fibromyalgia patients and 65 percent of all patients with chronic musculoskeletal pain use complementary therapies. Among fibromyalgia patients, three out of four have used herbs or lotions, 50 percent have tried spiritual healing, 40 percent have consulted with non-traditional health-care providers, and 30 percent have tried dietary interventions. Chiropractors, massage therapists, and acupuncturists were deemed the most helpful complementary health-care providers.

Currently, about 50 percent of all Americans use complementary therapies to treat various medical symptoms. In 1997, there were more visits to alternative care providers than to family doctors. Americans spend 15 billion dollars on alternative therapies, and most of this expenditure cannot be reimbursed.

There is no agreed definition of what constitutes complementary or alternative medical practice. Alternative treatments fall outside the realm of typical medical practice. Of course, the treatments this includes are in constant flux. Meditation and acupuncture are still considered alternative in some circles, but are part of conventional health care in much of the world. Some forms of alternative therapy, such as aromatherapy, therapeutic touch, colonic irrigation, magnets, and homeopathy remain extremely controversial. Many of the stress-management techniques such as meditation, biofeedback, and hypnosis are still considered alternative therapies, but now are often recommended by doctors.

The most prevalent alternative therapies are dietary, herbal, or nutritional in nature. Diet has played an important health role throughout history. Certain diets or fasts have been advocated for medicinal as well as religious purposes. Hippocrates wrote, 'There are certain persons who cannot change their diet with impunity; if they make any alteration for one day, or even part of a day, they are greatly impaired thereby.' There has been more written about dietary therapies for fibromyalgia and CFS than any other form of treatment.

Jane had tried all forms of dietary manipulation in treating her IBS and fibromyalgia. She was told that she was allergic to wheat, corn, pork, oranges, milk, eggs, peanuts, sugar cane, and food extracts. These were all gradually eliminated from her diet. There are no scientifically controlled data that would back up claims that this would help in treating fibromyalgia. It is possible that the elimination of certain foods or the addition of others could be beneficial. For example, milk and turkey are rich in tryptophan, which is metabolized to serotonin. Greater ingestion of tryptophan-rich foods might be useful to augment the body's serotonin stores. Becoming sleepy after drinking a glass of milk or following Christmas turkey may relate to the effects of raising serotonin levels. The countless books and recipes advising specific dietary treatments for fibromyalgia and chronic fatigue are based on such anecdotal information. However, no specific dietary alterations have been proven useful in fibromyalgia and CFS. The best thing you can do is to eat sensibly, avoid caffeine and alcohol for at least six hours before bedtime, and try eating small meals or snacks rather than two large meals. Keep a record of foods that upset you and avoid them. Your doctor should be able to refer you to a professional dietician.

No one had more experience with non-traditional treatments than Andrea. She had been using herbal remedies for years, following the recommendations of a naturopath. Each morning Andrea gobbled handfuls of vitamins and supplements, including echinacea, St. John's wort, ginkgo, kava root, ginseng, and shark cartilage. She told me that St. John's wort and echinacea gave her more energy. She wasn't sure about the others.

Herbs include any plant or plant product such as a root or fruit that is used for medicinal purposes. In the sixteenth century, botanical gardens and their medicinal herbs flourished on the grounds of medical schools. By the early nineteenth century, herbal medicine was dismissed as quackery and rarely practised in the United States. However, it never lost its status in Eastern medicine.

During the past thirty years, there has been an explosion of herbal therapy around the world. Currently there are more than twenty thousand herbal products available in the United States. The sale of herbs for medicinal purposes in the United States amounts to 1.5 billion dollars per year. Herbs are the largest growth area in retail pharmacy, far greater than the growth of conventional drugs.

Echinacea is the top-selling herbal remedy. A daisy-like flower, it is swallowed in a liquid form or sipped as a tea. Anecdotes suggest that it boosts the immune system. Advertising claims that it diminishes the severity and duration of colds and flus. A recent study did not support that claim, although it is safe and has been widely used throughout the world. St. John's wort, another herbal product, is available as a dietary supplement. It has been found to have antidepressant effects similar to the SSRIs. In Germany, St. John's wort has become the antidepressant of choice, out-selling Prozac seven to one.

Ginkgo biloba is derived from the ginkgo tree, which has been around for 300 million years. Chemical constituents of ginkgo affect platelets and free radicals that are important in blood flow. Ginkgo promoters claim it improves memory and energy related to these molecular actions. Kava root, obtained from a pepper plant found in the South Pacific, is said to induce a state of relaxation. It has been used to treat anxiety and as a muscle relaxant. Ginseng is manufactured from plants that grow wild throughout the world. Some come from China and some from the United States. Ginseng manufacturers claim that it improves oxygen utilization and decreases build up of lactic acid. This, too, is said to bolster immunity.

Andrea told me: *I am allergic to just about every medication. Everything that they have tried has made me sick. I am going to stick with only natural things from now on.* Andrea's naturopathic physician promoted the idea that natural products such as herbs were safe. On the wall of his office was a plaque proclaiming that 'herbs are God's way to cure disease.' He had told Andrea that the medical establishment discourages the use of herbs because pharmaceutical firms don't profit in their production. Andrea was told that the herbs' efficacy in fibromyalgia *were backed by scientific studies,* but the few studies that I was able to find were anecdotal, without a shred of valid evidence.

Why have these natural products become so popular? Patients with chronic illnesses want to be more proactive and have a greater role in their health. Herbal therapies allow them to do that. Because of their marketing as supplements, we don't think of them as medications. Every supermarket and health-food store has large sections with hundreds of products which are claimed to prevent all manner of ills. People can select herbal medications in their health-food store or their pharmacy without the inconvenience and cost of seeing health-care professionals. Natural, plant products are perceived to be safer and healthier than synthetically manufactured drugs. Religious beliefs may foster this notion. A thousand years of using herbs for medicinal purposes is reassuring.

People forget that 30 percent of all pharmaceuticals are derived from plants. These include digoxin, colchicine, codeine, taxol, and aspirin. Many consumers are not aware that most supplements and herbs contain synthetic ingredients. In fact, herbal or over-the-counter remedies can be dangerous. One of my fibromyalgia patients died from complications of taking tryptophan. In the 1980s, tryptophan was very popular as a natural amino acid that would help sleep, energy, and muscle pain. An impurity in the manufacturing process of tryptophan caused a systemic disease called eosinophilia-myalgia syndrome. Thousands of patients were severely impaired from this scleroderma-like disease. The herbs chaparral and comfrey have caused fatal liver damage. Ma huang, which contains the stimulant ephedra, has caused high blood pressure and heart attacks. Many herbs and natural products adversely interact with prescription drugs. Patients often do not discuss alternative treatments with their doctors. It was important that I knew that Andrea was taking St. John's wort. Because St. John's wort has antidepressant properties as well as side effects similar to SSRIs, I would not want Andrea taking them together.

In the 1980s, use of herbs and nutritional products was carefully scrutinized by the United States government's Food and Drug Administration (FDA). But in 1994, Congress passed the Dietary Supplement Health and Education Act; this allows dietary products and supplements to remain on the market unless there is clear proof that they harm people. Supplements only need to meet manufacturing standards of food products, far less stringent than drug manufacturing standards. Dietary supplements do not require proof of their effectiveness or of their safety. A specific disease cure cannot appear on their label, but herbal products and supplements may claim positive effects for a variety of symptoms.

Because the FDA does not oversee quality control, nutritional supplements or herbs may vary greatly in their purity or quality. In one study, the actual amount of St. John's wort varied from 20 to 90 percent of what various manufacturers had claimed was in their product. Some herbal preparations contain other ingredients such as heavy metals, which have caused dangerous reactions.

Andrea asked my opinion about the herbal products that she was using to treat her fibromyalgia and CFS. I told her that most of these supplements were harmless, but I could not attest to their efficacy. Before I recommend any treatment, I want to see scientifically reliable studies. I was also concerned about potential side effects and interactions with other medications. Fortunately, there are now a number of organizations and Web sites that can help doctors and their patients to explore the medicinal use of herbs. The FDA sponsors the MedWatch programme, and there are a number of herbal information centres on the Internet, including one site sponsored by the American Botanical Council.

Andrea was wearing magnets around her back and in her shoes. She recalled that when she first applied the magnets, *I laid on the floor and put one of the magnets under my mid-back. The magnets worked. I got a tingling sensation and when I got up, the muscles in my shoulders and neck felt less stiff.* Magnets are said to work by changing the magnetic field around our bodies. The delivery of electromagnetic fields to biological systems is the principle behind a number of techniques such as therapeutic ultrasound and transcutaneous electrical nerve stimulation. There is no evidence that the static magnets that Andrea was using could reduce pain. No sound research has proven that magnets work in any chronic illness.

Andrea had also been using homeopathic remedies as prescribed by her naturopath. Homeopathic medicine was developed by a German physician, Samuel Hahnemann, in the late eighteenth century. It is based on remedies that reproduce a person's symptoms when that specific substance is administered to a healthy individual. This is the principle of 'similars.' The medication must fit the specific pattern of symptoms for each individual. The other principle involved in homeopathy is that these medications will retain their activity even if they are repeatedly diluted. In fact, the more the substance is diluted, the more effective they are supposed to be. This is counter to every scientific principle. Homeopathic medications are serially diluted to thousands of parts of water. This would result in little if any original molecules of the starting substance, making doctors wary of homeopathic drugs.

Despite scientific scepticism, homeopathy has re-emerged in the West, buoyed by the explosion of interest in complementary medicine. In the United States, there were over 5 million visits to homeopathic providers in 1995, and the number of patients using homeopathy has increased five-fold in the last seven years. Authors such as Andrew Weil have touted its virtues. The popularity of homeopathy in the eighteenth century was largely a result of the ineffective and often barbaric practices of traditional medicine such as bloodletting. At least homeopathy caused no harm. With the scientific breakthroughs of the twentieth century, homeopathy fell into the category of placebo or quackery. Drugs such as penicillin and surgical procedures provided specific cures. Homeopathy is now being investigated in a rational fashion. There have been a number of clinical trials of homeopathy, including two in fibromyalgia, that have yielded mixed results.

Andrea wanted to stick with natural therapies. Much of the appeal of complementary medicine relates to the public's mistrust of science and technology. We constantly hear that additives, fumes, and toxins surrounding us are harmful. Alternative therapies get us 'back to nature.' The health-food movement preaches the superiority of natural ingredients. Herbal, nutritional, and vitamin therapies are advertised as totally safe.

Biomedicine is incomprehensible to most of us. It is impersonal. Complementary and alternative therapists offer a more personal approach to our health. There is more dialogue with the practitioner, more active participation in decision making. Therapies are in general tailored to the individual. Conventional medicine has focused almost exclusively on the physical aspects of disease. Alternative medical therapy is viewed as more holistic. In addition to these appealing virtues, complementary medical therapies have been extremely well marketed. Physician authors like Andrew Weil, Deepak Chopra, and Bernie Siegel have become celebrities as they promote natural ways to better health.

Alternative medical therapies are selected most often when traditional treatment has been ineffective. Complementary treatments are especially appealing to people with chronic illnesses such as fibromyalgia. Their medical condition is not life threatening, so people feel comfortable in experimenting and finding out what works best for them. The standard medications and the other traditional treatments used in fibromyalgia are often ineffective or create unpleasant side effects. Patients with fibromyalgia and CFS are primed to jump onto the bandwagon of unproven remedies. Those fibromyalgia patients who had the poorest health status and were most dissatisfied with their care were the most likely to use complementary treatment.

Experience, conviction, and anecdotal reports, not scientific studies, back up most claims made by complementary therapies. The most persuasive reports are published in books and magazines for the public. They have not been subjected to peer review. Many alternative medicine advocates claim that their treatments cannot be scientifically tested. This defensive posture can't be defended.

Pharmaceuticals and traditional forms of medical treatments must pass the rigour of randomized, controlled, scientific studies. A drug is compared with a placebo and specified outcome measures are evaluated with a blinded assessment. The public deserves that same scrutiny for complementary and alternative treatments. In the United States, the National Institutes of Health, in 1992, established an Office for the Study of Alternative Medicine in order to bring science to the field. Sophisticated chemical and pharmacological analysis of the active ingredients in herbal remedies is available and should be used before they appear in the marketplace. Just as with any new medication, the safety and efficacy and appropriate dose of alternative or natural treatments should be demonstrated before the public is exposed to them. Claims for efficacy should be supported by randomized, controlled, clinical trials.

The boundary dividing conventional and alternative medicine is often hazier than we are led to believe. Much of this division is based on arbitrary judgments regarding the role of specific and non-specific therapies. Traditional medicine seeks indisputable evidence that a specific intervention results in a specific outcome. Complementary therapy is less interested in cause and effect. This brings us to the subject of the placebo effect.

Placebo is Latin for 'I will please.' A placebo is any treatment that is either ineffective or has no known specific action on the condition being treated. Until the twentieth century, medical practice was virtually all placebo therapy. From ancient religious practices such as the laying on of hands, to Native American medicine men bloodletting, medical treatments had no definable symptom-altering activity. But with twentieth-century medical advances, specific treatments became available. New methodology was able to differentiate ineffective from effective therapies. In general, placebos are no longer prescribed to treat illnesses. 'Placebo' is now a pejorative term. Nevertheless, the placebo effect remains an integral part of any therapy.

Health-care providers have always utilized their status to influence patients. A doctor's zeal may result in public enthusiasm that is not scientifically justified. The doctor believes in their potions or pills. There is no intent to deceive. That is different from quackery. Many of the unproven remedies taken by people with fibromyalgia are recommended by well-meaning health-care professionals. Guaifenesin, magnesium, malic acid, and DHEA may eventually prove useful as there is some rational hypotheses behind their potential benefit. At this time, however, none of these treatments has been subjected to appropriate clinical trials.

Quackery relies on the placebo effect for fraudulent purposes. The word 'quackery' describes someone who 'quacks like a duck' about the virtue of unworthy therapies. In other words, a great deal of noise is made about nothing. Charlatans, a French word for 'faker,' and quacks have existed throughout medical history. Oliver Wendell Holmes observed, 'quackery and idolatry are all but immortal.' Some health-care providers are knowingly deceptive. From Denise's description of the medical tests ordered and treatments provided by her 'clinical ecologist,' I concluded that he was a charlatan. None of the tests on her blood, urine, or stool specimens was done in a reputable, accredited laboratory. The premise that she was infected with numerous microbes was based on fraudulent tests. She was also told that her blood levels of metals such as zinc and arsenic were dangerously high, but these test results were uninterpretable. Based on this dubious data, she received intravenous chelation to remove these heavy metals followed by intravenous vitamins and antibiotics to boost her immunity and cure the infections. There is no evidence that any of these therapies work. None was covered by her medical insurance plan and thousands of dollars were wasted.

Traditional medicine recognizes the power of the placebo effect. In general, a placebo will improve symptoms by approximately 30 percent in studies of most chronic illnesses, including fibromyalgia. Some argue that placebos have no place in modern-day medicine. Nevertheless, any new medication must be proven to be significantly more effective than a comparison placebo before the drug is approved by the regulatory authorities. This is the basis for all randomized, double-blind clinical trials. If not, the drug effect is considered to be non-specific, even if it was helpful.

In the broadest sense, much of what we do as doctors is non-specific and could be viewed as a placebo effect. Simply wearing a white coat and providing comfort is therapeutic. Touching a patient, whether by a doctor, a massage therapist, a chiropractor, or a religious adviser, elicits beneficial physiological effects. The basis of psychotherapy, counselling, and cognitive behavioural treatments is to attain general changes in mood and attitudes. These are non-specific, placebo forms of treatment that can be very effective.

Medicine does not need arbitrary divisions between mainstream and complementary treatments. Non-specific effects, whether from a pill or from touching and talking with our patients, can be therapeutic. The placebo effect is ubiquitous in medicine. Sir

William Osler recognized this, commenting, 'faith in the gods or in the saints cures one, faith in little pills another, hypnotic suggestion a third, faith in a plain, common doctor a fourth.' Our only job is to determine what is effective versus not effective treatment. Any therapy that is effective should no longer be considered alternative.

FICTION

- **Alternative treatments are safer and more natural than medications.**

- **Complementary therapies can't be judged or evaluated like conventional treatments.**

- **Many foods cause pain and exhaustion because of subtle allergies and must be avoided.**

- **Placebos are useful for getting rid of bothersome patients.**

- **Herbs and nutritional therapies do not interact with medications.**

FACTS

- **Most forms of complementary treatments have not been adequately tested to know their efficacy or safety.**

- **Alternative treatments should be subject to the same rigorous standards as conventional medical therapies.**

- **There is no single diet or foods to avoid. Eat sensibly and nutritiously.**

- **Tell your doctor about complementary treatments. They may react adversely with medications.**

- Alternative or complementary treatments can be helpful adjuncts to conventional therapies.

- Both traditional and alternative medical therapies have powerful, non-specific, or placebo effects.

- Many complementary treatments will be proven effective over time and will no longer be considered alternative.

14

How Do I Find Accurate Information?

BECKY was referred to me by a specialist in internal medicine four years ago. As she sauntered into my office late one Friday afternoon, her broad smile and firm handshake were immediately engaging. Dressed plainly, wearing thick glasses with her hair pulled tightly into a bun, Becky's matronly appearance belied a warm and confident manner.

She had grown up in Massachusetts, the second of three children. Becky's father was a doctor and her mother, after raising the children, had completed a master's degree in health-care economics. Becky and her siblings each had been accomplished students and Becky had graduated from an Ivy League college.

Becky was unusually bright and insightful. She first became ill six years earlier when she was forty-three years old, working as a college professor. She described a very insidious onset of widespread muscle pain: *My muscles became increasingly sore and stiff. Every muscle began to tighten up. I couldn't get the knots out of my neck and back. My sleep became erratic and I was exhausted. Each afternoon I had to put my head down on my desk. It felt like my body was betraying me. I had never had a headache in my life. I had always felt indestructable.*

Becky's search for a medical diagnosis followed the frustrating trail of Patty and Denise. Multiple specialists were consulted and countless tests were ordered. Eventually, Becky's consultant suspected that she might have fibromyalgia and sent her to a rheumatologist. He agreed with that diagnosis. Becky recalled:

I was initially relieved when I was told that I had fibromyalgia. But the doctor couldn't tell me much about it. He couldn't tell me how I got it. He wasn't very encouraging either. He said that there was no effective treatment, but that I needed to start exercising, which seemed absurd since I could barely walk up the stairs. His parting remark to me was that I would just have to learn how to live with it.

I didn't find that very satisfying and turned to the Internet for more information. My education and background are in science and computers. I launched a personal campaign to learn everything I could about my illness. There were loads of sites on the World Wide Web about fibromyalgia. First, I reviewed those sponsored by doctors or medical professionals.

The Internet has become a powerful source of medical information to the public. At least 45 percent of Americans have access to the Internet and soon most will be regular visitors to the World Wide Web. There are more than 4 million medical or health-related documents on the Web. The Internet has allowed people to seek their own health information and to make better health-care decisions. Web sites devoted to particular illnesses have provided valuable information to patients and their families. On-line support groups promote self-help and emotional support.

However, there are many pitfalls when searching the Web for medical knowledge. Medical misinformation is especially pervasive on the Internet. There is little editorial or quality control on the Web. Unfiltered medical information may present a very unbalanced view of an issue. Anyone with a Web site can claim to be an expert. Most consumers do not have the scientific background to distinguish fact from fancy, or to know who is an expert and who is a quack. Sensational anecdotes abound on the Internet, especially in 'chat rooms.' It is hard to know if the Web site sponsor has a financial interest. Because the Internet is so difficult to regulate, it is easy to promote illegal, fraudulent, and harmful medical products and devices.

It is relatively simple to find medical information on almost any subject on the World Wide Web. It is much more difficult to know whether this information is credible. As a 1997 editorial in *JAMA* stated: 'The problem is not too little information, but too much, vast chunks of it incomplete, misleading or inaccurate . . . The Net, and especially the Web, has the potential to become the world's largest vanity press.' There are very few studies that have evaluated the reliability of medical information on the Internet. In contrast to peer-reviewed journal articles, there is no established format to evaluate the quality of information on the Net. Furthermore, the information is provided by and directed towards an eclectic group of health-care professionals, consumers, and business vendors.

Becky understood that much of this information was anecdotal and not necessarily credible. After all, anyone can set up a Web site. A $100 software package can convert any home PC into a Web server. It takes little skill to add sophisticated graphics and logos, making the site more official appearing.

Becky was told by many Web sites that fibromyalgia was a specific disease, capable of causing an infinite number of symptoms. One site declared, 'If you have fibromyalgia, looking both ways when going into traffic causes you to feel dizzy. You develop oesophageal reflux. You put on weight. Some objective signs are ridges on the fingernails, goose bumps behind the upper arms and thighs, and mottling of the skin. You are electromagnetically sensitive.' Becky wondered whether every unexplained medical symptom could be explained by fibromyalgia. Bloating, teeth grinding, dizziness, chronic ankle sprains, weak knees, weak ankles, leg cramps, allergies, gastritis, rashes, painful intercourse, and double vision were each attributed to fibromyalgia.

These all-embracing symptoms are not part of the fibromyalgia definition. Such sweeping, indiscriminate definitions obscure fibromyalgia as a useful diagnostic label. According to the symptoms attributed to fibromyalgia on many of the Web sites, fibromyalgia indeed was a 'dustbin diagnosis.'

Web sites told Becky that the medical profession would not take her complaints seriously. A fibromyalgia patient complained in a chat room, 'People with fibromyalgia are either brushed off like I was or told that it is all in their head. I began to worry myself sick. So many of us feel betrayed by the medical profession. I was determined to find doctors who knew exactly what was wrong.' So Becky tried to do just that.

One Web site, sponsored by a doctor who suffers from fibromyalgia, declared that fibromyalgia was caused by '. . . an accumulation in the muscle of toxic metabolic products which can be cured with guaifenesin. I will consider changing my medications, my physical therapies and my exercise routines, but I will not consider going without guaifenesin. You know it is working when your urine and sweat become dark and smelly. This indicates a release of waste, excess acids and toxins.'

Becky recounted: *I tried the guaifenesin, but I didn't feel any better. I got in touch with the doctor who recommended it. She suggested that I hadn't avoided some of the many substances that can block the effect of the drug. I spent the next six months following their suggestions, but I didn't see any improvement.*

There is a common theme on Web sites and in books that the medical profession hides crucial information and withholds breakthrough alternative therapies. People on self-help Web sites have reprimanded me for not recommending guaifenesin and other unproven remedies. Hillary Johnson, the American author and CFS patient, accused the researchers at the National Institutes of Health to be 'indifferent to the fate of scientists outside their institution who wish to be involved in the discovery process, and at worst, hostile to any scientific inquiry not their own.' She laments the national cover-up of CFS: 'The story of the American epidemic and the people whose lives it destroyed continue to play out in a kind of half-light, unseen and unfelt in most regions of the culture.'

We are inundated with the latest and greatest medical claims in every facet of the media. The Internet is just the newest and the most powerful source of medical information and misinformation. The media has a profound effect on our health. For many, the only contact with medical and scientific discoveries comes from what is read in the press or watched on television. A 1997 National Health Council survey found that television was the single most important source of medical news for Americans, ahead of advice from their doctors. Of Americans, 40 percent get most of their medical information from television compared with 36 percent from doctors. The information on fibromyalgia recently presented on national television has been as disconcerting as that found on the Internet.

The *20/20* segment regarding the role of brain surgery in fibromyalgia was exciting television, but poor medical journalism. Many of my patients were equally distressed following a *Dateline* article on fibromyalgia a few months earlier. The neurologist interviewed by Maria Shriver stated that fibromyalgia does not exist. In stark contrast to these remarks, Shriver then interviewed a fibromyalgia patient who had become devastated: 'There are days when she needs a cane or has to spend most of her time in bed. She is treated with excruciating shots deep into her sensitive tender points, and takes twenty-three pills a day to ease her pain, fight insomnia, and combat the depression that so often accompanies fibromyalgia.' Such a desperate patient makes dramatic viewing, but is not representative of people with fibromyalgia. No one pointed out that 70–80 percent of people with fibromyalgia work full-time and most take very few medications.

Media coverage of CFS has been equally misleading and sensationalized. CFS has been portrayed as a new, infectious disease of epidemic proportions. The 11 October, 1985 *Sacramento Bee* declared 'Mysterious Sickness Plagues North Tahoe.' A *Rolling*

Stone story in 1987 was titled 'Journey into Fear: The Growing Nightmare of Epstein-Barr Virus.' The cover of *Newsweek* on 12 November, 1990 declared 'Chronic Fatigue Syndrome. Mysterious Illness Afflicts Millions.'

I was amazed by the different focus of our Boston newspapers when reporting the Kevorkian suicide of the Massachusetts woman with fibromyalgia and CFS. One paper's headline exclaimed, 'Doctors say her case treatable, non-fatal.' Their account focused on whether physician-assisted suicide is morally justified when the potential suicide victim has a non-fatal disease. I was interviewed along with three other medical experts. A balanced, medically accurate description of fibromyalgia and CFS was provided. The less responsible news coverage was headlined, 'Docs clash over suicide, autopsy.' This story focused on the medical profession's inability to diagnose and treat disorders like CFS properly. Emphasis was on the frustration of patients and the futility of medical therapy. Two attorneys and one patient with CFS were quoted, but no medical experts. One story informed whereas the other sought to stir up the public.

Gulf War media coverage has been politicized and sensationalized. David first learned that illnesses were being linked to the Gulf War when he picked up the November 1995 issue of *Life* titled 'The Tiny Victims of Desert Storm: Has Our Country Abandoned Them?' The cover pictured Gulf War veteran Sgt. Paul Hanson with his three-year-old son, Jayce, born without arms or legs. The story described seven families whose children had birth defects and who claimed the cause to be exposure during the Gulf War, concluding, 'No one knows how many abnormal babies have been born to Gulf vets . . . many still question whether Defense Department scientists are really seeking the hard answers.'

Dr. Steven Joseph, then U.S. Assistant Secretary of Defense, accused the media of sensationalizing the Gulf War situation: 'I think the media in general did a very poor job . . . there was some rather cynical self-interest in some of the media approach . . . I think the *Life* piece was both a charade and very cynically done. . . . We talked to the people at *Life,* told them what the scientific data showed, and that within a week or two there would be a scientific journal article in the most prestigious medical journal in the country that showed there was no evidence for congenital defects, and asked them to delay publication until the scientific article came out, to balance their story with the information that was there. They went ahead and published it in the most sensationalistic way anyway. I think that did a great disservice to not only people who served in the Gulf, but to their families. I think they scared a lot of people. There was no basis, no scientific, factual basis for their story. It was just a cover and a headline and I think represents the worst kind of journalism.'

Potential Gulf War poisons made powerful television drama. Dan Rather stated, 'The veterans may be suffering side effects from experimental vaccine . . . Approximately two thousand soldiers could be victims of what doctors call a "multiple chemical sensitivity syndrome."' Although the overwhelming medical opinions were that the vaccines and medications did not cause Gulf War syndrome, the media quoted a few scientists who voiced the opposite opinion.

The vets and their families suffered greatly from media misinformation. Many still believe that they were poisoned by chemical weapons. We all watched as the Gulf War unfolded on CNN. We heard the alarms going off and the soldiers putting on gas masks. Imagine how they felt. The media reinforced the vets' worst fears about toxins. Some delayed having children because of the reports of birth defects. Vets' wives and children started to come down with similar symptoms. The majority of the media coverage ignored the scientific and medical reports in favour of controversy and hype. Speculation took the place of science. Anecdotal stories convinced some that a toxin had made them ill, and the government was covering it up.

It was impossible not to be swayed by the media frenzy. James Hale, a marine employed in the Gulf, said: '. . . it wasn't until that stuff came up in the news and you started seeing it repeatedly that you started thinking, you know, you get an ache, where did that come from . . . and then all of a sudden on TV people were getting sick, people were having this problem, babies are being born with deformities, and everybody started linking it to the war. And that's when you start, wow, thinking . . . maybe there is something out there and you start wondering about yourself and then every little illness that you start wondering about . . . I think the American public loves a good mystery . . . it sort of feeds on it.'

The media coverage of medicine is often sensationalized and misleading. Journalists use terms such as 'the newest,' 'biggest,' or 'fastest.' We hear reports of 'wonder drugs,' 'cancer break-throughs,' and 'arthritis cures.' A medical reporter knows that weak headlines don't sell. Fresh and dramatic medical news sells. Studies that were touched upon months ago are 'old hat.'

The public is especially vulnerable to media hyperbole when it comes to illnesses like fibromyalgia and CFS. These disorders are filled with uncertainty. The less science knows about an illness, the more misinformation the public receives. People like Becky became prey to false hope and radical cures.

Becky made a survey of the fibromyalgia remedies marketed on the Internet. Some sites used blatant emotional claims to sell a product. One Web site featured Dominie, who descibed her fifteen-year battle with fibromyalgia. She had been in constant pain until 'In May of 1996, something happened that would change my life completely. Through my research on the Internet, I learned about OPCs (olgomeric proanthcyanidins). I found out that these nutritional antioxidants from France are totally safe and had produced stunning health results across Europe for over a decade. Not only did they help fibromyalgia, its free radicals fight to prevent stroke, heart attacks, and cancer. Since starting to use OPCs, I feel like my life has been given back to me.' Using the 1-800 number provided, the magical OPCs could be ordered over the Internet for only $45.50 for sixty tablets.

Becky eventually set up her own Web site for fibromyalgia information. I agreed to serve as a medical advisor. Like other doctors, I have trouble keeping up with my own patients' inquiries let alone trying to tackle those of strangers. However, I recognized the need for sound medical information about fibromyalgia and related illnesses on the Internet.

Becky found 150 sites on the World Wide Web dedicated to fibromyalgia. Of these, 50 percent were sponsored by a single person with no health-care background. Another 25 percent were sponsored by organizations or products with a financial interest in fibromyalgia. Becky and I established a rating system to evaluate the reliability of the medical information provided by each site. Less than 30 percent of the sites had any accurate medical information. The vast majority were either selling products or featured someone talking about their own trials and tribulations with fibromyalgia.

Many of these Web sites depicted a sad and hopeless situation. One proclaimed: 'Fibromyalgia is an invisible disease. It gains strength inside your body by attacking anywhere it pleases. Like a tainted candy chocolate, it looks delicious on the outside, but the inside is filled with the poison of confusion and agony. Fibromyalgiacs have everything taken away from them in just a moment of time. It rips you apart, piece by piece, it takes no prisoners.' As if that wasn't depressing enough, the person finished by saying 'Most of all, it brings to mind an unspeakable thought of suicide. Fibromyalgiacs are drowning.'

Becky's Web site was up and running during the same week the *20/20* programme on brain surgery for the treatment of fibromyalgia was aired. Becky was inundated with requests for information from fibromyalgia patients throughout the U.S. She responded that there was not a shred of proof that such surgery works in most people. Becky interviewed a number of prominent neurosurgeons, who expressed grave concern that this surgery was performed on 'desperate people, eager to obtain any sort of relief that might be offered them. They are easy prey to someone who offers them a quick fix when there is no quick fix.' Since that programme Becky has disseminated the results of the study that found spinal stenosis or Chiari malformation to be no more common in people with fibromyalgia than in healthy control patients.

Becky has accepted the limitations of our medical knowledge. She wants information to be as reliable as possible and doggedly pursues balanced and honest information for herself and for other people. This takes dedication. It is easy to succumb to the arrows of unbridled zeal, self-interests, and power struggles. A number of reliable Web sites devoted to fibromyalgia information are listed on pages 233–234.

It will continue to be difficult for people to wade through the morass of medical misinformation on the Internet and in the media. The best approach is to discuss new medical information with your health-care professionals. Bring in written material that you have come across. Write down your questions, no matter how trivial they may seem. In the future, doctors need to do a better job of providing the most accurate information and education to their patients and to the public.

FICTION

- Fibromyalgia Web sites are of good quality.

- Chat rooms are a healthy way for people to communicate.

- Most books about fibromyalgia are written by medical experts.

- Americans get most of their medical information from their doctors.

FACTS

- There is little editorial or quality control on the Web. Unfiltered medical information may present a very unbalanced view of an issue.

- Chat rooms can provide a sense of community, but beware of misinformation and self-interests.

- Conditions such as fibromyalgia, CFS and Gulf War syndrome are prone to receive inaccurate reporting since they are so controversial and there are very limited scientific facts.

- Media coverage of medicine is often misleading and sensationalized.

- Be cautious when medical claims ignore or attack scientific studies.

15

How Do I Find the Right Doctor and Support?

PATTY, Denise, and Becky all bounced back and forth from doctor to doctor, searching for the correct diagnosis and treatment. Most people tell me that it took a number of years to be diagnosed with fibromyalgia. Doctors exclude diseases. We are good at ruling out dangerous disorders, but not good at understanding many common illnesses. When repeated examinations, X-rays, and blood tests are normal, we reassure patients that there is nothing to worry about. But that strategy backfires when we attempt to relieve our patients' anxiety. When no disease can explain symptoms, doctors conclude that the person is actually healthy, but one of 'the worried well.' Often a psychiatric consultation is recommended, which frequently causes the patient to become angry and defensive.

The rheumatologist that Becky saw made the correct diagnosis of fibromyalgia. He examined her carefully and ordered all of the appropriate laboratory tests to exclude any other disease. His advice to Becky, however, was, 'You have got to learn to live with it.' There was no treatment plan or follow-up appointments. Becky wasn't satisfied. She sought more advice and more information. So she turned to the Internet and found a Web site that provided fibromyalgia patients with what was claimed to be 'The Good Doctor List.' She sought out one of these doctors, who came highly recommended.

This naturopathic doctor had published a book claiming that his remedies could cure fibromyalgia and CFS. The book received widespread praise from patient support groups. Becky followed his complicated, therapeutic protocol, which included guaifenesin, nutritional treatments, hormones, antifungals, antiparasitics, and a mixture of pain relievers, antidepressants, and eye drops. Intravenous chelation therapy was used to rid her body of metabolic toxins. After two months of these treatments she felt no better. Because none of this expert treatment was covered by Becky's health insurance, she was $5,000 poorer.

Becky and Denise had logically concluded that the doctors who were recommended on these 'Good Doctor' lists would be recognized authorities on CFS and fibromyalgia. However, the recommendations were from patients, not from other doctors or medical groups. Very few of the listed doctors had done any research on fibromyalgia or CFS. None of them had published their findings in peer-reviewed journals. Certain fibromyalgia and CFS patients recommended these doctors because of their personal attributes, not their medical credentials.

Some of the qualities of these self-proclaimed fibromyalgia and CFS experts were commendable. Becky extolled that the holistic expert was compassionate: *he listened to me*. Nothing is more important in achieving an effective doctor-patient relationship. These 'Good Doctors' also uniformly practised or recommended alternative and complementary forms of health care. That is reasonable, provided standard treatment isn't neglected. But Becky became concerned that some of the good doctor's claims were too good to be true. Becky said, *He told me exactly what was wrong and explained how he would treat it. There was no discussion of my background, my interests, or my personal life. When his treatments weren't working, he suggested a totally new group of remedies.*

At that second visit, Becky was also given a form to complete designed to assist her in receiving disability coverage. The phone number and the fax number of a lawyer 'specializing in assuring that patients with fibromyalgia and chronic fatigue syndrome receive adequate compensation' was provided. Becky questioned the relevance of this since she was working and had no plans to stop working. The furthest thing from her mind was disability.

Patients with fibromyalgia and CFS face a dilemma. Either they can continue to work despite pain and limitations, choose to modify their work schedule, or quit altogether. If they choose the latter, they often step down the slippery slope of the current medical-legal compensation system in the United States. Focus then switches from recovery to causation, injury, and disability. During the past century, conditions variously called repetitive strain injury, writer's cramp, railway spine, and telegraphist's wrist have linked a self-reported injury to chronic illness. Mercury poisoning from dental fillings, electromagnetic fields, carbon monoxide, fumes from sick buildings, or exposure to video display terminals have each been postulated to cause chronic illnesses like fibromyalgia and CFS.

A growing number of fibromyalgia patients have been involved in disability proceedings. This creates a moral dilemma for doctors. Doctors are not trained to evaluate the role of workplace activities on a person's level of pain or to judge a person's physical capabilities. In a biomedical disease model, the doctor might be able to estimate the level of pain and disability following an injury, such as a fractured leg. However, in conditions such as fibromyalgia, the doctor has no objective criteria to base such judgments on. Disability in chronic back pain or in fibromyalgia is based on a disease model, but there is no known disease. Doctors are asked to judge a person's ability to walk 50 feet or lift 50 pounds. This has no relevance to fibromyalgia. We can only guess what the long-term problems will be in people with chronic illnesses. A court or insurance company usually appoints a medical examiner who has never treated the patient, but provides 'independent' confirmation. This system cannot fairly judge an illness that is based on symptoms. We must rely totally on the patient's assessment of their pain and suffering.

Jon, as do many people with fibromyalgia and chronic back pain, filed for occupational compensation because his pain did increase after he fell at work. The U.S. insurance system fosters such action. Jon, like most Americans, had been led to believe that back pain is caused by an injury or abnormal physical stress on the spine. The television blasts forth commercials from lawyers (often called 'ambulance chasers') that assert 'You are entitled to compensation after your accident. Call me no matter how trivially you think you were hurt.' Unfortunately, Jon's suffering worsened after the disability determination process began. He described his frustration during the litigation hearings: *I feel like someone is always watching me. My lawyer tells me that if I do any part-time work, I will ruin my chance of getting long-term disability coverage. Some of the doctors think that I'm not trying hard enough to get better. The insurance company thinks I'm faking. What a joke! All I want is to be whole again – I want to go back to work.*

Once a person stops working, pain and function seldom improve, and often worsen. If you have to prove that you are ill, you can't get well. An adversarial, medical-legal debate generates frustration and anger. This is the reason why I discourage my patients from litigation. Nevertheless, doctors must recognize that injuries and the workplace can contribute to chronic pain. Work environment changes, short-term disability, and employee-employer flexibility go a long way to prevent long-term work loss. In some situations, compensation is required, and I will be the patient's advocate. In my practice, only 10 percent of fibromyalgia patients have stopped working. However, 30 percent have needed to make some job modifications. The long-term outcome of patients with chronic pain, be it back pain or fibromyalgia, is better when patients return to a productive existence. The medical profession must work with patients, claimants, insurance companies, and society to promote rehabilitation, self-care, and a return to work.

Becky continued to teach despite her fibromyalgia. She understood the limitations of our medical understanding of chronic illnesses and the ill-conceived notion that they must be cured. Many
patients are angry and frustrated when I admit to not knowing a
cure. They want to get 'fixed' and be 'like I used to be.' But,
chronic illness is rarely curable. I teach my patients that we can all
feel better *despite* being ill. Becky just needed a plan to get started.

Start with a family doctor who will coordinate your medical
care. You should feel comfortable talking about anything with
this doctor. Your family doctor should know you as a person and
be interested in you.

Using my father's American football analogies, your family
doctor should be the quarterback who lines up the players on your
treatment team. Obstacles abound however. Many general practitioners are not familiar with fibromyalgia. Some do not want to
deal with any functional or mind–body illnesses. You need to
discuss this openly. Your doctor does not need to be a fibromyalgia
expert. But he or she needs to be open to the construct of fibromyalgia. He should be receptive to discussing it, not disparaging of it.

Fibromyalgia treatment requires time. The managed health-
care system in the United States insists that patient encounters be
infrequent and brief. Health insurers reward quick diagnoses, not
lengthy health-care discussions. In general, the major incentive
under managed care is to 'do less.' Managed care often misman-
ages people with chronic illness. Illnesses like fibromyalgia run
counter to any cost-cutting measures. Fibromyalgia therapy is
prolonged, often lifelong. People need extra time from their family
doctor, just when managed care experts are exerting pressure to
shorten office visits. The 'target' at the largest health maintenance
organization in New England is for the doctor to see eighty
patients per week. This results in a maximum of ten to fifteen minutes of time per patient.

No matter what the medical problem, such pressure results
in dissatisfied patients and harried, frustrated doctors. There is
precious little time to probe the unique personality and psycho-

social issues of each patient. No time is available to provide information and education to patients and to their families. Doctors are not reimbursed for patient education. Nowadays, family doctors are penalized for 'excess' utilization of consultants. Family doctors have become triage officers, deciding who to refer and when. Referrals are often primarily based on economic decisions. Chronic illnesses like fibromyalgia are best treated when multiple, health-care professionals pool their talents.

The family doctor should be able to exclude the presence of other medical and surgical disorders. He or she should be comfortable with providing psychological and rehabilitative advice. Most health-care visits should be to the family doctor. The role of the specialist is to advise the family doctor and to help in the management of patients with treatment-resistant fibromyalgia.

Specialized care for people with fibromyalgia is best handled by a rheumatologist or a rehabilitation specialist (see Table on Treatment, page 134). Such a doctor should have significant experience and expertise in treating the disorder. The initial evaluation by the fibromyalgia specialist should include a thorough review of the available clinical records, a detailed medical history, a physical examination with special attention on the joints and tender points, as well as a neurological examination. The patient should be asked how the symptoms began, how they impact on life and work, what aggravates the symptoms, what makes them better. Inquiring about mood, stress, and sleep is essential. When appropriate, a more detailed sleep questionnaire, a psychiatric history, and a mental status examination should be performed. Activity and exercise levels should be evaluated. All current and prior medications must be documented, including alternative and non-prescription items.

Laboratory tests should be kept at a minimum and might include a blood count, thyroid function test, and an erythrocyte sedimentation rate. Screening tests, such as for a connective tissue disease or Lyme disease, are to be discouraged unless there is clinical suspicion of those diagnoses. MRIs and CAT scans are rarely necessary. Indiscriminate fishing for a missed diagnosis leads to more unnecessary tests.

Deciding on initial treatment involves assessment of information and education about the illness and all potential therapies. Pharmacological therapy and non-medicinal treatment should be discussed. A copy of all recommendations should be sent to the family doctor. Appropriate follow-up should be arranged. Often a person with fibromyalgia will only need to see the specialist once or twice each year. Most of the plans can be carried out by the patient with their family doctor.

Coordinated, team care for fibromyalgia is expensive (see Table on Treatment, page 134). There is no reimbursement for education or information sessions. Insurance cover for physical therapy or physiotherapy is usually limited. There is little, if any, insurance coverage for group or individual exercise programmes. Managed care preaches holistic medicine. But when it comes to chronic illness like fibromyalgia, there is no coverage for prolonged, individualized therapy, exactly what people with chronic illness need. This makes it virtually impossible for any single health-care professional to spend enough time with a patient.

Mental health coverage is inadequate, especially for talk therapy. In her book *Welcome to My Country,* Lauren Slater notes: 'Especially in this time of managed care, more emphasis seems to be placed upon medication and the quick amelioration of symptoms, short-term work and privatized, profit-making clinics, than upon the lovely and mysterious alchemy that comprises the cords between people, the cords that soothe some terrors and help us heal.'

How do you find a fibromyalgia expert? Hopefully, your family doctor will be able to refer you to a specialist who treats many patients with fibromyalgia. Most communities have a rheumatologist. Of course, as Becky learned, not every rheumatologist has an interest in taking care of people with fibromyalgia. In the United States, the local chapter of the Arthritis Foundation provides lists of such individuals. When initially scheduling an appointment to see a rheumatologist or rehabilitation specialist, ask their office if the doctor treats fibromyalgia on a regular basis.

No matter whom you see, you must feel confident. During my own illness, I went to every expert in Boston. 'Expert' doctors are usually defined by the prestige of the medical schools they attended, the number of research publications they have churned out, and the number of diplomas and citations on their consulting room walls. Certain magazines and books honour such doctors and you can easily access lists such as 'The Best Doctors in America.' I am on this list and I am proud of that, but I know how fickle such lists are. Academic credentials have no relationship to a doctor's humanism or humility.

Initially, I unsuccessfully sought out a doctor who could help me. Eventually, I found two doctors who helped guide me. They worked with me as partners in my recuperation. Neither has published much in medical journals, nor trained at a world-class hospital. But, they both are healers. Mike, my family doctor, is a solo practitioner, nowadays a rarity. His surgery is a chaotic mess, with books, journals, and papers scattered everywhere. Nick, my psychiatrist, shares modest consultation space with a large number of other mental health professionals. Neither Mike nor Nick are physically imposing. They don't blow you away with a command of the medical literature or a list of their achievements. They both have a quiet, interactive style. I sense their compassion. I know that they are interested in me, not just my illness. Both Mike and Nick recognize the limitations of medicine. They recognize that doctors often don't have all the answers.

Denise was disappointed that I could not tell her why she had become chronically fatigued. I offered to help lessen her symptoms, but could not provide a cure. The ecologist doctor she consulted told Denise that her immune system was poisoned and that he could cleanse it. This would cure her. When it didn't, she became more distraught. The chiropractor told Jonathan that multiple spinal subluxations caused his back pain and his fibromyalgia. Manipulation would fix it. It didn't. Telling people that we have the answers may generate initial patient confidence, but eventually will add to peoples' despair.

You and your doctor should be partners in your care. Traditionally, doctors have taken a paternal approach to patients. Many doctors fear that patients lack the medical knowledge and perhaps the strength or good sense (especially when sick or in pain) to make rational health-care decisions. But, the days of doctors playing God are over.

Some very concerned and competent doctors are simply not interested in treating fibromyalgia or other chronic health disorders. They prefer a different type of challenge. The rheumatologist Becky consulted dutifully excluded all 'serious' illness and then dismissed her with a pat on the head. Such doctors may be excellent problem solvers, but not good listeners or healers.

Doctors, as well as patients, vary greatly in their capacity to accept medical uncertainty. Medical students and young doctors are not trained to handle the uncertainty of most illnesses. It is important that the vagaries of fibromyalgia be discussed with candour. Most of my patients have readily accepted the ambiguities of fibromyalgia. I don't pretend to know how to fix it. My patients and I grapple with the obscurity and perplexity that surrounds fibromyalgia. Many doctors fear that being open about their lack of understanding fibromyalgia will erode their patient's confidence. Some patients do respond best to an authoritarian, omnipotent doctor. Such patients are usually quite passive and inflexible regarding their health. The typical person that I treat wants their doctor to be a partner rather than a boss.

Be wary of technocrats, doctors who order every conceivable test on you. Very few tests are necessary for the diagnosis of fibromyalgia. You may end up having unwarranted procedures. With today's focus on biotechnology, the art of medicine has become an afterthought. Doctors rely increasingly on tests and machines rather than on human contact. CAT and MRI scans, lasers and laparoscopies are powerful diagnostic tools, but they tell us little about pain and suffering. Expensive and invasive tests have no place in the management of most of the common illnesses like fibromyalgia, CFS, or headaches.

You also must find support from your family and friends. It is often especially difficult for a spouse or family members to empathize with fibromyalgia patients. People look better than they feel. Medical sceptics abound. Denise's recovery wasn't complete until her husband became involved. Poorly understood illnesses such as fibromyalgia isolate people. Loneliness adversely affects our recuperative power. Express yourself to others. If you find this difficult, write it down. There have been numerous studies demonstrating that writing about illness improves recovery. I have certainly found that true and have used writing as my catharsis.

Support groups can be very helpful if they truly support people. Unfortunately, sometimes they degenerate into gripe sessions. Such support groups are often dominated by individuals who feel victimized and wronged by society. Medical information can be one sided or incorrect. A highly charged political and social atmosphere interferes with the best intentions of support groups and patient advocates. Health-care professionals are often depicted as either friends or foes. Balance is lost. There is no middle ground. The potential danger of support groups is exemplified by certain Lyme disease groups with 'self-taught medical experts who considered themselves victims of a corrupt scientific establishment . . . and which organized its own scientific conferences, financed its own research, created its own scientific publication, and trumpeted its own medical experts.' I have witnessed attacks on investigators such as Dr. Steven Straus by certain CFS organizations, and now Dr. Allen Steere by Lyme disease groups.

Our fibromyalgia treatment programme brings six to ten patients together once a week for ten weeks (see Table on Treatment, page 134). Health-care professionals are always present. The focus is on achieving wellness rather than a cure. One of the benefits of bringing a number of patients together is watching the friendships that form. A number of my patients have generated their own informal support networks. There is also a list of fibromyalgia and CFS support groups available through national organizations (see Web sites additional resources, page 233). Any programme that truly supports patients provides them with a sense of control and independence.

More family doctors are becoming knowledgeable about fibromyalgia. Most rheumatologists, rehabilitation specialists, and physiotherapists treat fibromyalgia patients every day. Therefore, it should not be difficult for you to find a caring and compassionate family doctor and an experienced specialist. Work with a doctor who is flexible and tolerant. Find someone who gets to know you and who will accept who you are. It may take some searching to find the right person, but they are out there.

FICTION

- **Everyone with fibromyalgia should be treated with 'natural' supplements, such as magnesium, malic acid, DHEA, and guaifenesin.**

- **If you are in too much pain or too exhausted to work, find a lawyer to help you get appropriate compensation.**

- **Your doctor should exclude every disease possibility before considering the diagnosis of fibromyalgia.**

- **If your doctor can't explain exactly what is wrong with you, find another who can.**

- **Most fibromyalgia patients do not need to consult with a mental health professional. If you are told to see a psychiatrist or to take antidepressants, the doctor thinks that it is all in your head.**

- **Support groups are essential to your recovery.**

FACTS

- Misinformation about this illness is rampant. There is no single best or essential treatment.

- Once people stop working, their symptoms generally worsen.

- Your family doctor should be able to eliminate potential diseases with a careful history, physical examination, and simple laboratory tests.

- Your doctors should be your partners in finding the best treatment for you. No one has all the answers, but you and your health-care professionals need to be flexible and try different approaches.

- Taking care of chronic illnesses like fibromyalgia requires a lot of time. It is labour intensive.

- Rheumatologists and physiatrists (rehabilitation specialists) tend to be the most knowledgeable fibromyalgia specialists. A consultation with a psychiatrist or psychologist is often helpful.

- Support groups must truly support people and should include advice from a health-care professional. Complaining, griping, and finding fault will only increase distress.

- Fibromyalgia is often best treated by a multidisciplinary team of health-care providers.

16

Will I Get Better?

THE word *doctor* derives from Latin *docere,* to teach. My most important accomplishments have been as a teacher. During the first twenty years of my professional career, I taught medical students and trainees in internal medicine and rheumatology. During the past decade, my teaching has been predominantly to my fibromyalgia patients. I believe that education is the cornerstone of effective treatment.

I give each new fibromyalgia patient a detailed lecture, cramming as much information as I can into an hour. I initially focus on the differences between diseases and illnesses. Disease is defined in terms of biological and structural abnormalities in the organs of our body. Diseases are determined by dysfunction of these organs and are called 'organic.' Illness is each person's perception of feeling unwell. Illness is a departure from wellness and may be present without organic disease. Fibromyalgia is an example of such an illness. Some people may be afflicted with diseases such as diabetes or cancer, yet feel well. Illness cannot be measured objectively. It does not necessarily correlate with structural or objective phenomena.

We next talk frankly about the limitations of the term 'fibromyalgia.' I discuss the concern whether the diagnosis of fibromyalgia is enabling or disabling. Steve, a patient of mine who lives in Maine, wrote a letter to the editor in response to Dr. Groopman's article in *The New Yorker*: *In your article on fibromyalgia in the November 13 issue, author Jerome Groopman presents the views of Harvard psychiatrist Dr. Arthur Barsky, who contends that 'even honoring this bundle of symptoms with a medical label may be doing more to make people sick than to cure them.' This is directly counter to my experience as a person who was diagnosed with the syndrome seven years ago. I had spent a scary and confusing two years dealing with pain and what is referred to as fatigue, but would be better described as a total depletion of the will. During this time, I underwent examinations to establish whether I had Lyme disease, osteoarthritis, lupus erythematosus, multiple sclerosis, a spinal tumour, or other debilitating diseases. I was seriously relieved to find that I suffered from a recognized syndrome that had been named and is being investigated by the medical community. I was informed at the time that the symptoms were real, but the illness was not degenerative and in fact no pathology could be identified at this time. Far from causing me to become trapped in the belief that my future held only 'debility and doom,' as Dr. Barsky claims, I was given the information that I needed to proceed with my life. Exercise was highly recommended and I was encouraged to remain active despite the feedback I was getting from my body.*

Without a diagnostic label for fibromyalgia, CFS, and IBS, I would not be able to educate and inform my patients. In my clinic and in my research, I need to operate with a discrete diagnosis. My patients need a name for their illness. Yet, if the labels are used for political or social-economic decisions, they can be disabling. The misuse of terms like 'ruptured disc' and 'whiplash' have led to a cottage industry of disability and compensation that has bankrupted companies and disabled patients.

We must be flexible enough to discard these arbitrary diagnostic boundaries when exploring the pathophysiology of chronic pain and fatigue. Illnesses such as fibromyalgia and CFS are best understood from a bio-psychological, rather than a biomedical framework. These conditions are neither physical or psychological, but both. The ancient Greeks and Romans believed that the mind and body were intimately linked together. Hippocrates, the father of medicine, wrote about the healing harmony of psyche and soma in the fourth century B.C.

That all changed when Descartes and other scholars of the 1600s, as well as Western religions, fostered the idea that the church or the spirit was separate from the state or the body. For the next three centuries two principles dominated the Western biomedical model. The first principle, called 'reductionism,' taught that all illness has a single cause with a specific outcome. The second principle of 'dualism' has taught that illness is either organic or functional.

George Engel, a professor of both medicine and psychiatry, was one of the most persuasive advocates for an integrated mind-and-body illness model. His bio-psychosocial model of the 1970s proposed that diseases and illnesses result from simultaneously interacting biological, environmental, and personal factors. We now recognize that every 'psychological disorder' has biological influences, and vice versa.

A mind *and* body illness model is more personal and more flexible than the traditional mind *or* body model. Artificial boundaries, such as disease or illness, mental or physical, mind or body, dissolve. Illness is appreciated as a personal experience. Wellness and illness are points on a continuing spectrum. The boundaries between health and illness become less distinct.

A bio-psychological illness paradigm allows my patients to recognize illness factors that they can modify in contrast to those that are fixed. Sarah no longer shouldered blame and guilt for being depressed. She accepted that genetic and biological factors predisposed her to depression and fibromyalgia. Jon and Denise stopped searching for a cause and a cure. Chronic illnesses are not caused by a single physical or psychological event. Physiological changes discussed throughout this book connect the mind with the body. Fibromyalgia, chronic pain, fatigue, headaches, IBS, and depression can only be understood if patients and doctors are comfortable with these new bio-psychological models of illness. The brilliant neurologist Charcot said in 1889, 'Disease is very old and nothing about it has changed. It is we who change as we learn to recognize what was formerly imperceptible.'

After fibromyalgia, the illness that I treat most commonly is rheumatoid arthritis. As early as 1909, research suggested that anxiety and worry provoke rheumatoid arthritis. During the next century, rheumatoid arthritis was often classified as a psychosomatic disease. However, shortly thereafter, the mechanisms of inflammation and immunity that drive rheumatoid arthritis were elucidated. Rheumatoid arthritis was now a purely 'physical' disease. There was no reason to focus on its psychological aspects.

Ironically, as the basic biological understanding of rheumatoid arthritis has recently exploded, there has been a simultaneous resurrection of interest in its psycho-social factors, especially stress. The most important outcome variables in rheumatoid arthritis, or in fibromyalgia, are psycho-social. These include levels of education, income, work status, and concurrent mood disturbances. Prior depression and chronic stress are important factors in predisposing people to rheumatoid arthritis as well as to fibromyalgia. Each of these factors is very important in determining how people respond to their chronic illness.

Genetic illness factors can not be modified. But, our response to any illness can be modulated. Catastrophizing over chronic illness is especially destructive. The heart attack patient may change his habits when it comes to smoking and lack of exercise, for instance, or may become paralyzed by fear and uncertainty. After my brain surgery, I learned firsthand about the adverse influence of catastrophizing. Jon had put himself into a similar frame of mind. He felt helpless and rejected. Virginia told me that I was her last hope.

Even the anticipation of pain and distress creates changes in the brain's blood flow and decreases immune function. In contrast, humans can be conditioned to enhance their immune system. Just as the lupus mice were conditioned to develop a positive immune effect from sugar water even when not receiving the immunosuppressive medication, patients with chronic illnesses have improved their immunity following psychological conditioning techniques such as group therapy. People can change negative thoughts. Mental health professionals and other stress management psychologists teach patients to cope better. Hopelessness and helplessness are replaced by realism and cautious optimism. If people begin to take charge of their health, they can do a lot for themselves.

There will be times when our symptoms inexplicably worsen. Much of the ebb and flow of fibromyalgia can be traced to how we handle stress. Therefore stress-management techniques become an important focus of treatment. Scott's stress often triggered a migraine headache. The frequency and severity of his headaches and his neck and shoulder pain diminished dramatically with meditation and relaxation exercises. Many of my patients find these stress reduction techniques helpful. We can learn to control our illness rather than let it control us.

We cannot optimally adapt to an illness if we are occupied in blaming others. Jonathan blamed the fall at work for his misfortunes. Denise blamed undetected viruses and sick building fumes. David blamed toxins from the Gulf War. Because we do not know the cause of fibromyalgia, blame is a useless practice. Blaming things outside of ourselves can be comforting because it gets us off of the hook and we don't have to take responsibility for our conditions. But, it also distances us from the only illness factor under our total control, our emotions. While we sink in the midst of our pain and suffering we become angry and we feel victimized. We look for someone to blame. People often ask 'Why me?'

The Dalai Lama wrote, 'This kind of thinking poses hidden dangers. If we think of suffering as something unnatural, something that we should not be experiencing, then it's not much of a leap to begin to look for someone to blame for our suffering. If I am unhappy, then I must be the victim of someone or something – an idea that's all too common in the West. The victimizer may be the government, the educational system, abusive parents, a dysfunctional family, the other gender, or our uncaring mate. Or we may turn blame inward: there is something wrong with me, I am the victim of disease, of defective genes perhaps. But the risk of continuing to focus on assigning blame and maintaining a victim stance, is the perpetuation of our suffering – with persistent feelings of anger, frustration and resentment.'

What is the best approach when people are convinced that their pain and suffering were caused by a physical event beyond their control? I tried to give Jon and David a balanced and non-judgmental medical opinion. First, people must recognize that injuries and trauma rarely 'cause' chronic pain. The fractured leg heals. The neck injury fades away. Persistent structural changes in the body rarely follow mild or modest injury. Nevertheless, medical, media, and legal systems promote the misconception that injuries are responsible for most chronic pain and therefore someone else is responsible. In general, blame promotes anger. When our lives are dominated by seeking retribution, we can't get on with the process of living our lives to the full.

The most essential lesson for my patients is that they can get better. In fact, almost everyone gets better if they work hard at it. Some fibromyalgia 'opponents' state that rheumatologists like me have been able to do very little for our patients. They point to studies from fibromyalgia centres that demonstrated no significant change in symptoms after seven years. In *The New Yorker* article, Dr. Groopman quoted Dr. Bohr, who said 'these people are not being helped.' Groopman commented '. . . many doctors were also gloomy about the long-term prognosis for fibromyalgia sufferers: the published data on patients who have been cared for in speciality rheumatology clinics and have received the usual combination of psychiatric medication, analgesics, and stretching exercises – have been extremely discouraging. And yet the same doctors regularly refer patients to clinicians like Dr. Goldenberg. They are ready to forego the income and passively endorse the generic programme in order to park the patient with someone who believes in the malady and is willing to oversee a condition that is not likely to improve.'

I disagree. Fibromyalgia is a very treatable illness. Studies from Australia and Canada have found that fibromyalgia patients in the community, not attending speciality clinics, had an excellent prognosis. After two years, 50 percent of those patients had a complete remission of their symptoms without taking any drugs. Many people with chronic illnesses such as fibromyalgia never reach specialists like me. Their symptoms are mild and often remit spontaneously. As with headaches or fatigue, many of us have transient fibromyalgia symptoms that do not require significant medical attention.

Most fibromyalgia outcome studies are conducted at specialist referral centres such as mine. Patients in these speciality clinics tend to have the most treatment-resistant symptoms and a poorer prognosis than people in the population at large. That doesn't mean the situation is hopeless. We have followed our patients in Boston carefully for twenty years. Although most patients continue to have some fibromyalgia symptoms, 70 percent are better than when they were first diagnosed. Of our fibromyalgia patients, 75 percent feel 'well' or 'very well' on most days. Almost all are working. It is important that we dispel any notion that fibromyalgia, whether in the community or in speciality clinics, carries a very poor prognosis.

When patients have not improved with simple management and seek the advice of a specialist, a multi-disciplinary therapeutic approach should be provided (see Table on Treatment, page 134). Our fibromyalgia treatment team includes a rheumatologist, a physiatrist (rehabilitation specialist), and sometimes a psychiatrist. The rehabilitation specialist makes specific recommendations for physical therapy and may also suggest acupuncture, chiropractic, or various forms of neuromuscular treatment. Our rehabilitation specialist performs trigger point injections, although rheumatologists and neurologists are also trained to do that. If concurrent depression or anxiety is present, I recommend a consultation with the psychiatrist. The psychiatrist helps manage complicated drug regimens. Individual or group counselling, such as in our cognitive behavioural and stress reduction programme, is often helpful in coping with chronic illness. Counselling might be handled by a psychologist, a social worker, a nurse, or by clergy. Specialists in pain management can be invaluable in those patients who fail standard analgesic therapy. Rarely, an inpatient care setting in a pain unit or rehabilitation hospital is necessary.

Although medications and physical treatments are never curative, they are very helpful. As discussed in the previous chapters, specific therapies must be tailored to each person. That means that I first need to know the individual. I need to understand how each patient has been dealing with his or her illness. Some of us live better with our symptoms than others. The doctor who told Becky that she needed to learn to live with her symptoms was right. But he did not teach her how to do that. That is what I try to do.

Every person has a unique personality. Each of us handles our symptoms differently. There is no cookbook therapeutic recipe. That is why I spend so much time trying to listen to my patients and get them to understand themselves better. Only when I know the person, can I prescribe that individual's best treatment. A 'patient-centred' rather than a 'doctor-centred' plan works best.

For some patients, a simple explanation of fibromyalgia will alleviate most of their worries. Others may need much more attention from a number of different health-care providers. The diagnostic criteria for fibromyalgia, CFS, and IBS provide a uniform framework for making a diagnosis. However, such criteria tell us nothing about how that illness affects each individual. I evaluate each patient to determine which symptoms are most important to that individual. Only at that juncture will I be able to tailor the individual treatment to that person.

Some of my colleagues ask me how I can tolerate treating so many people with chronic, unexplained illnesses such as fibromyalgia, CFS, back pain, and headaches. The perception by much of the medical profession is that such patients are very frustrating. They don't get better and often they don't really want to get better.

None of these perceptions is true. I find that taking care of people with fibromyalgia is very rewarding. There are some people who are so locked into their world of suffering that I have not been able to help them. This is uncommon. For many, small gains occur over months or years. Spontaneous remissions and exacerbations are the rule. Gradually, I have returned to the reason that I chose medicine for a career: to make a difference, on a person-to-person basis. I know every patient who I see can feel better. But it takes hard work.

The great majority of people tackle their illness and adversity with great harmony. Every person with a chronic illness must make some adjustments. Wishing or waiting for it to go away doesn't work. Taking a proactive role in finding the best approach to better health does work. Most fibromyalgia patients lead a full and active life. Achieving balance while we are ill requires practice and patience. Keeping things in perspective in the face of illness and uncertainty is no easy task. The most important lessons that I have learned from my patients, my wife, and my own illnesses are found on these pages. I hope they will allow you to better balance the scales of your own illness.

FICTION

- There is little that you can do other than accept the pain.

- Fibromyalgia never gets better, only worse over time.

- There is no effective therapy.

- Fibromyalgia may lead to diseases like multiple sclerosis or lupus.

- Most people with fibromyalgia become disabled.

FACTS

- Learning about your illness and how to understand yourself better is essential for your health. What works for one person may not work for another. You must take charge.

- There will be ups and downs, often aggravated by stress. We can change the negative reactions to our illness. Catastrophizing and blaming are unhealthy.

- Getting better is hard work, but we each can do it.

- Fibromyalgia never becomes another disease.

- Fibromyalgia may go away, but we need to be very proactive, not wait around passively in the hope that it will. With appropriate information and treatment, everyone should feel better.

EPILOGUE

PATTY and I have made important changes in response to our experience with chronic illness. Facing a medical crisis forced us both to examine what was most important in our lives. Always worrying about what other people thought, I had to be the best doctor, father, and athlete in others' eyes. Now, I concentrate more on what life means to me.

Many patients have told me that their illness made them a stronger and happier person. That is certainly my experience. I feel more at peace with myself. Everything seems more meaningful. Before our illnesses, Patty and I did not have the depth of caring and togetherness that we now share. Each day is more precious. My family, my friends, and my work are most important to me. A few years ago I got all pumped up after being interviewed on *Good Morning America*. The same feeling happened recently when I was on *Today*. That elation lasted just a few days and left me with an empty feeling. Fame is fleeting. A permanent, much deeper joy comes from holding Patty, my children, and my grandchildren.

Andrew Weil describes sickness as a step towards health. The two states are relative: one cannot exist without the other. Patty and I cherish our health much more after experiencing illness. I ask my patients to learn from their illness because illness is a powerful teacher. It forces change. It makes us more flexible. No one wants to get sick, but it happens to each of us.

Patty and I have learned to accept what we can't change, and to change things that are under our power. We recognize that a lack of control does not mean 'giving up' or taking a fatalistic outlook. People cannot control their health any more than their lives. Bad things happen to each of us that are beyond our control. But people are amazingly resilient and can bounce back from the gravest misfortune.

Once we understand ourselves better, we can face adversity with more equilibrium. Quick cures, hidden secrets, or the all-knowing guru seldom provide the way to better health. Staying in focus, finding your equilibrium, and getting to know yourself does. The better we know ourselves the more we can change. We must accept some uncertainty. Better health does not require having all the answers.

Lewis Thomas observed people's growing health obsession: 'All sorts of things seem to be turning out wrong, and the century seems to be slipping through our fingers here at the end, with almost all of our promises unfulfilled . . . but I can think of one thing that is wrong with us and eats away at us: we do not know enough about ourselves. We are ignorant about how we work, about where we fit in, and most of all about the enormous, imponderable system of life in which we are embedded as working parts. The only solid piece of scientific truth about which I feel totally confident is that we are profoundly ignorant about nature.'

I have learned to seek support from others, especially from my family and friends. I always wanted to appear cool, calm, and collected – self-sufficient. Medical training reinforces the virtues of detachment. Doctors are taught not to get too involved with their patients. The 'best' (or 'easiest') patients are the ones that never complain. The last thing that I wanted to do was to complain, to cry out for help. Spiro and Mandell, who wrote the book *When*

Doctors Get Sick, said 'the powerlessness and loneliness of patienthood remind sick doctors of what in health we may have given up: close relationships.'

Patty has always been much more open with her feelings than me. Denial wasn't ingrained in her personality. She always gave to others and in turn was able to profit from their love. I have learned to be open and to demonstrate my feelings. Many of us withdraw from our feelings so that we won't get hurt. That robs us of the depth of love and caring that provides meaning to our lives.

Illness forces us to find better balance in our lives. The caduceus, the emblem of a physician, depicts the opposing forces of good and evil. Two snakes are entwined on the caduceus rod, heads facing in perfect alignment. Hippocrates taught that health is forged by balancing the forces of the mind and body.

Finding my own balance has never been easy for me. Like many of my patients, I always focused on what I was not getting done, rather than what I was doing. As a metaphor for my personal life, I have always thought that I had poor hand-eye coordination. Whether trying to stay upright on a balance beam in high school, taking dancing lessons with Patty, or hitting a golf ball, I always felt tentative. Instead of trying for better balance I became more tenacious. I would just try harder. For most of my life, exercise was an obsession. If I went a single day without my usual, intense workout, I felt tired and blue. However, all the fun from exercise that I knew as a boy had long since evaporated. I would push through the exercise routine like a robot, not knowing exactly what I was doing or why I was doing it.

Sometimes when I am at the health club, I see that frenzied look on the faces of people trying desperately to exercise away their pain and suffering. Like everything else that is 'good for you,' exercise can also be bad for you. I often see people exercising 'through the pain,' causing further pain and possible injury. Now, I pay more attention to why and how I am exercising.

Learning to let go is important. Professional athletes talk about being in a zone, trusting their instincts, going with the flow. Qi or 'energy flow' is at the heart of Eastern culture and medicine. I have learned to do a yoga stretch without worrying that I will fall on my face. I calm my breathing, focus my eyes ahead, slowly bring my arms to the side, and then stand on one foot. I'm getting better. I'm working hard to achieve better balance as a doctor, a husband, a father, and a grandfather. It takes practice and patience.

If our minds are cluttered with worry and anticipation, we can't become one with the sport, our work, or with our illness. We can't find a flow. I now sometimes feel that effortless flow. I can sense my muscles and tendons as they respond to stretching. Friends who paint or write tell me the same thing. You can best enjoy the activity, the process itself, once you become one with it.

It holds true in illness. Unless you find balance in your health and your illness, you will suffer unduly. Watching Patty, Denise, Jonathan, Becky, and thousands of my fibromyalgia patients overcome their illness has been inspiring. Each learned how to balance their lives and their illness. The lessons that I have learned from fibromyalgia have served me well, as a doctor, as a patient, as a husband, as a father, and as a grandfather. Writing them down is the most important thing that I have done. It is my way to thank my wife and my patients, who have been my teachers.

NOTES

PREFACE

ix. I was interviewed by Katie Couric on the 10 January, 2001 *Today* show, and in 1992 on *Good Morning America*. My research on fibromyalgia has been featured in *The New York Times* on 7 September, 1989 and 1 August, 2000 and *The Boston Globe* on 25 January, 1988 and *Boston Herald* on 27 June, 1999. The article 'Hurting All Over' by Dr. Jerome Groopman published in *The New Yorker* magazine, pp. 78–92, on 13 November, 2000, explored the many controversies surrounding fibromyalgia. Dr. Groopman not only spent months talking to experts on both sides of this issue, he also spent time with me in my office and observed as I saw patients.

x. See *Hippocrates, Ancient Medicine,* Loeb Classical Library, Harvard University Press, 1984, vol. 1. Hippocrates in the fourth century B.C. set the stage for exploring the relationships of mind to the body.

CHAPTER 1

3, 4. M. Yunus, et al. 'Primary fibromyalgia (fibrositis): clinical study of 50 patients with matched normal controls.' *Semin Arthritis Rheum* 11:151–171, 1981. This report by Dr. Muhammed Yunus and colleagues was the first review of fibromyalgia to appear in a peer-reviewed rheumatology journal.

5. Valleix's quote from, M. D. Reynolds. 'The development of the concept of fibrositis.' *J Hist Med Allied Sci* 38:7, 1983. This is one of a number of excellent reviews on the medical history of fibromyalgia. For more on the history of fibromyalgia, see also R. M. Bennett. 'Fibrositis: misnomer for a common rheumatic disorder.' *West J Med* 134:405–13, 1981.

6. W. R. Gowers. 'Lumbago: Its lessons and analogues.' *Br Med* 1:117–21, 1904. This treatise on back pain describes the characteristic symptoms of fibromyalgia.

6. R. Stockman. 'The causes, pathology and treatment of chronic rheumatism.' *Edinburgh Med J*; 15:107–16, 1904. Osler quote from Reynolds, 1983. The pivotal studies of Kellgren and Lewis are found in, J. H. Kellgren. 'Observations on referred pain arising from muscle.' *Clin Sci* 3:175–190, 1938.

7. J. G. Travell and D. G. Simons. *Myofascial Pain and Dysfunction: the Trigger Point Manual,* Baltimore: Williams & Wilkins, 1983. Travell's work popularized the idea that trigger points represented specific anatomic abnormalities. Also see C. Z. Hong and T. C. Hsueh. 'Difference in pain relief after trigger point injections in myofascial pain patients with and without fibromyalgia.' *Arch Phys Med Rehabil* 77:1161–66, 1996; C-Y J. Hsieh, et al. 'Interexaminer reliability of the palpation of trigger points in the trunk and lower limb muscles.' *Arch Phys Med Rehabil* 81:258–264, 2000.

7. E. W. Boland. 'Psychogenic rheumatism: the musculoskeletal expression of psychoneurosis.' *Ann Rheum Dis* 6:195–203, 1947. Most medicine and rheumatology textbooks in the 1950s through the 1970s included a chapter entitled 'psychogenic rheumatism' that focused on fibromyalgia.

8. F. Wolfe, et al. The American College of Rheumatology 1990 criteria for the classification of fibromyalgia: 'Report of the Multi-centre Criteria Committee.' *Arthritis Rheum* 33:160–172, 1990. Fibromyalgia was defined as widespread chronic pain involving all four quadrants of the body and the presence of at least 11 of 18 tender points. These criteria have been useful to classify patients providing some uniformity for clinical studies.

9. M. Martinez-Lavin, et al. 'Fibromyalgia in Frida Kahlo's life and art.' *Arthritis Rheum* 43:708–9, 2000. Kahlo's 1944 self-portrait *The Broken Column* depicts arrows piercing her body at sites of tender points. It is proposed that she had fibromyalgia.

9, 10. Prevalence and incidence of fibromyalgia in the population, see K. P. White, et al. 'The London fibromyalgia epidemiology study: the prevalence of fibromyalgia syndrome in London, Ontario.' *J Rheumatol* 26:1570–76, 1999; T. Schochat, et al. 'The epidemiology of fibromyalgia.' *Br J Rheumatol* 33:783–786, 1994; K. O. Forseth, et al. 'A population study of the incidence of fibromyalgia among women aged 26–55 years.' *Br J Rheumatol* 36:1318–23, 1997. The incidence of fibromyalgia has varied widely in certain countries and ranges from 1 to 5 percent of the population. Fibromyalgia is the second most common rheumatic illness, after osteoarthritis. For discussion of fibromyalgia developing in certain illnesses and at different ages, see G. D. Middleton, et al. 'The prevalence and clinical impact of fibromyalgia in systemic lupus erythematosus.' *Arthritis Rheum* 37:1181–1188, 1994; D. Buskila, et al. 'Assessment of nonarticular tenderness and prevalence of fibromyalgia in children.' *J Rheumatol* 20:368–370, 1993. Fibromyalgia has been reported following hepatitis, parvovirus, HIV infection, and Lyme disease and is more prevalent in people with chronic inflammatory diseases such as rheumatoid arthritis or SLE than in the general population.

10. The role of muscle in fibromyalgia, see R. W. Simms, et al. 'Lack of association between fibromyalgia syndrome and abnormalities in muscle energy metabolism.' *Arthritis Rheum* 37:794–800, 1994; N. J. Olsen and J. H. Park. 'Skeletal muscle abnormalities in patients with fibromyalgia.' *Am J Med Sci* 315:351–58, 1998. MRI spectroscopy demonstrated no major metabolic muscle abnormalities in a series of fibromyalgia patients matched for activity levels to controls. Some minor changes have been reported in muscle fibre reactivity and muscle relaxation. Also, see A. Hakkinen, et al. 'Strength training induced adaptations in neuromuscular function of premenopausal women with fibromyalgia.' *Ann Rheum Dis* 60:21–26, 2001. Isometric muscle strength in women with fibromyalgia was comparable to that of healthy females.

10, 11. For further discussion of the hormonal pertubations in fibromyalgia, see I. J. Russell. 'Advances in fibromyalgia: possible role for central neurochemicals.' *Am J Med Sci* 315:377–84, 1998; P. S. Hench. 'The ameliorating effect of pregnancy on chronic atrophic (infectious rheumatoid) arthritis, fibrositis, and intermittent hydrarthrosis.' *Proc Staff Meet Mayo Clin* 13:161–167, 1938; A. Korszun, et al. 'Follicular phase hypothalamic-pituitary-gonadal axis function in women with fibromyalgia and chronic fatigue syndrome.' *J Rheumatol* 27:6:1526–1530, 2000; P. H. Dessein, et al. 'Hyposecretion of adrenal androgens and the relation of serum adrenal steroids, serotonin and insulin-like growth factor-1 to clinical features in women with fibromyalgia.' *Pain* 83:313–319, 1999; S. R. Pillemer, et al. 'The neuroscience and endocrinology of fibromyalgia.' *Arthritis Rheum* 40:1928–39, 1997. Research demonstrates that corticotropin releasing hormone (CRH) and the autonomic nervous system are important in understanding the symptoms of fibromyalgia. Also, see D. Buskila, et al. 'Assessment of nonarticular tenderness and prevalence of fibromyalgia in hyperprolactenimic women.' *J Rheumatol* 20:2112–15, 1993; E. Toussirot, D. Wending. 'Fibromyalgia after administration of gonadotropin-releasing hormone.' *Clin Rheumatol* 20:150–2, 2001.

11. Potential genetic aspects of fibromyalgia are reported in M. B. Yunus, et al. 'Genetic linkage analysis of multicase families with fibromyalgia syndrome.' *J Rheumatol* 26:408–12, 1999; D. Buskila, et al. 'Familial aggregation in the fibromyalgia syndrome.' *Semin Arthritis Rheum* 26:605–11, 1996; L. T. H. Jacobsson, et al. 'Low prevalences of chronic widespread pain and shoulder disorders among the Pima Indians.' *J Rheumatol* 23:907–9, 1996. M. Offenbaecher, et al. 'Possible association of fibromyalgia with a polymorphism in the serotonin gene regulatory region.' *Arthritis Rheum* 42:2482–88, 1999. This report demonstrated that a specific serotonin receptor gene was more common in fibromyalgia than in normal women.

11, 12. Moldofsky's initial description of the sleep disturbances in fibromyalgia can be found in H. Moldofsky, et al. 'Musculosketal symptoms and non-REM sleep disturbance in patients with "fibrositis syndrome" and healthy subjects.' *Psychosom Med* 37:341–351, 1975. A recent study by his group suggests that there are different alpha intrusion patterns and a phasic form of alpha sleep activity correlated best with fibromyalgia symptoms: see S. Roizenblatt, et al. 'Alpha sleep characteristics in fibromyalgia.' *Arthritis Rheum* 44:222–230, 2001.

12. D. L. Goldenberg, et al. 'A randomized, controlled trial of amitriptyline and naproxen in the treatment of patients with fibromyalgia.' *Arthritis Rheum* 29:1371–1377, 1986. In the early 1980s we compared standard anti-inflammatory doses of naproxen, 500 mg twice daily, with low doses of amitriptyline, 25 mg at night, in people with fibromyalgia. The amitriptyline was superior to naproxen, which was not much better than placebo in treating the symptoms of fibromyalgia. D. L. Goldenberg, et al. 'A randomized,

double-blind crossover trial of fluoxetine and amitriptyline in the treatment of fibromyalgia.' *Arthritis Rheum* 39:1852–59, 1996. More recently we combined amitriptyline at night with low doses of Prozac in the morning. Both amitriptyline and Prozac were better than placebo in treating the symptoms of fibromyalgia. However the combination of 20 mg of Prozac in the morning with 25 mg of amitriptyline at night was significantly better than either medication alone.

12, 13. G. K. Adler, et al. 'Reduced hypothalamic-pituitary and sympathoadrenal responses to hypoglycemia in women with fibromyalgia syndrome.' *Am J Med* 106:534–543, 1999; L. J. Crofford and M. A. Demitrack. 'Evidence that abnormalities of central neurohormonal systems are key to understanding fibromyalgia and chronic fatigue syndrome.' *Rheum Dis Clin N Am* 22:267–284, 1996; L. J. Crofford. 'Neuroendocrine abnormalities in fibromyalgia and related disorders.' *Am J Med Sci* 315:359–66, 1998; E. N. Griep, et al. 'Function of the hypothalamic-pituitary-adrenal axis in patients with fibromyalgia and low back pain.' *J Rheumatol* 25:1374–81, 1998. Drs. Adler, Crofford, and Griep have been studying the neuroendocrine aspects of fibromyalgia. Their findings have demonstrated that alterations in the hypothalamic-pituitary-adrenal system are important in many aspects of the fibromyalgia syndrome. In fibromyalgia, chronic stress may trigger a resetting of the control of hormones such as CRH and noradrenaline.

13. For studies on growth hormone, see R. M. Bennett, et al. 'Low levels of somatomedin-C in patients with the fibromyalgia syndrome: a possible link between sleep and muscle pain.' *Arthritis Rheum* 35:1113–1116, 1992; R. M. Bennett, et al. 'Hypothalamic-pituitary-insulin-like growth factor-I axis dysfunction in patients with fibromyalgia.' *J Rheumatol* 24:1384–9, 1997. Rob Bennett was the first to report that about 25 percent of fibromyalgia patients have low levels of insulin-like growth factor. Following growth hormone replacement, fibromyalgia symptoms and tender points improved: see R. M. Bennett, et al. 'A randomized, double-blind, placebo-controlled study of growth hormone in the treatment of fibromyalgia.' *Am J Med* 104:227–31, 1998.

13. Research regarding the autonomic nervous system in fibromyalgia, see D. J. Clauw, et al. 'Heart rate variability as a measure of autonomic function in patients with fibromyalgia and chronic fatigue syndrome.' *Arthritis Rheum*

38 R25, 1995; H. Cohen, et al. 'Autonomic dysfunction in patients with fibromyalgia.' *Semin Arthritis Rheum* 29:217–27, 2000. Involvement of the sympathetic nervous system is associated with orthostatic intolerance, cardiac irregularities, and exaggerated vasomotor responses.

CHAPTER 2

16. D. L. Goldenberg. 'Fibromyalgia syndrome: An emerging but controversial condition.' *JAMA* 257:2782–2787, 1987. For quote from Groopman, see *The New Yorker* 2000, pg. 90.

17. H. Dinerman, et al. 'A prospective evaluation of 118 patients with the fibromyalgia syndrome: prevalence of Raynaud's phenomenon, sicca symptoms, ANA, low complement, and Ig deposition at the dermal-epidermal junction.' *J Rheumatol* 13:368–373, 1986. Certain features of fibromyalgia may mimic a systemic connective tissue disease. However, fibromyalgia essentially never turns into a systemic connective tissue disease. Many patients with connective tissue diseases do have symptoms of fibromyalgia.

19. D. L. Goldenberg, et al. 'High frequency of fibromyalgia in patients with chronic fatigue seen in a primary care practice.' *Arthritis Rheum* 33:381–387, 1990. We assessed patients diagnosed with CFS blindly to see whether they fitted the diagnostic criteria for fibromyalgia. Of the CFS patients, 70 percent had the necessary tender points and the typical symptoms of fibromyalgia. Every patient with CFS who reported that they were having muscle pain was found to have fibromyalgia.

20–22. For critiques of the concept of fibromyalgia, see M. L. Cohen and J. L. Quintner. 'Fibromyalgia syndrome, a problem of tautology.' *Lancet* 342:906–909, 1993; T. Bohr. 'Problems with myofascial pain syndrome and fibromyalgia syndrome.' *Neurology* 46:593–597, 1996; N. M. Hadler. 'Fibromyalgia, chronic fatigue, and other iatrogenic diagnostic algorithms.' *Postgrad Med* 102:161–77, 1997; (contains the quote on page 21 from Hadler). The quote from Dr. Thomas Bohr is from the transcript of the 4 Jan, 2000 *Dateline* programme. He stated that doctors and support groups exacerbate the disorder by convincing patients that they are invalids with an incurable problem. Dr. Bohr described that lawyers who sue for large disability payments encourage patients not to be actively treated.

21, 22. For this quote from Dr. Fred Wolfe, see Groopman, *The New Yorker* 2000, pg. 89.

22. R. B. Haynes, et al. 'Increased absenteeism from work after detection and labelling of hypertensive patients.' *N Eng J Med* 299:741–44, 1998. The labelling of patients as hypertensive resulted in increased work absenteeism. If a label is not applied appropriately, a patient may consider himself or herself more fragile and adopt a sick role. Also, see P. Brown. 'Naming and framing: the social construction of diagnosis and illness.' *J Health Social Behavior* 11:34–52, 1995.

22–24. For more debate regarding the utility of a fibromyalgia diagnosis, see M. O. Makela. 'Is fibromyalgia a distinct clinical entity? The epidemiologist's evidence.' *Baillieres Clin Rheumatol* 13:415–419, 1999; I. J. Russell. 'Is fibromyalgia a distinct clinical entity? The investigator's evidence.' *Baillieres Clin Rheumatol* 13:445–454, 1999; K. P. White, et al. 'Does the label "fibromyalgia" alter health status and function?' *Arthritis Rheum* 43 (suppl 9): S12, 2000.

24. Differences among doctors' and patients' perception about CFS are described in A. Deale, et al. 'Patients' perceptions of medical care in chronic fatigue syndrome.' *Soc Sci Med* 52:1859–64, 2001; M. Stevens, et al. 'General practioners' beliefs, attitudes and reported actions toward chronic fatigue syndrome.' *Aust Fam Physician* 29:80–5, 2000; S. W. Twemlow, et al. 'Patterns of utilization of medical care and perceptions of the relationship between doctor and patient with chronic illness, including chronic fatigue syndrome.' *Psychol Rep* 80:643–58, 1997.

CHAPTER 3

28. Groopman J. *Second Opinions.* Viking, New York, 2000. Pg. 4

29. For Gowers's description of lumbago, see Gowers, 1904.

29–31. For update on current concepts of chronic back pain, see R. A. Deyo and Y. J. Tsui-Wu. 'Functional disability due to back pain. A population-based study indicating the importance of socioecenomic factors.' *Arthritis Rheum* 30:1247–1253, 1987; D. J. Clauw, et al. 'Pain sensitivity as a correlate of clinical status in individuals with chronic low back pain.' *Spine* 24:2035–2041, 1999; K. C. Wachter, et al. 'Muscle damping measured with a modified pendulum test in patients with fibromyalgia, lumbago, and cervical syndrome.' *Spine* 21:2137–42, 1996; S. J. Atlas, et al. 'Long-term disability and return to work among patients who have a herniated disc: the effect of disability compensation.' *J Bone Joint Surg* 82:A4–15, 2000.

31–33. For in-depth discussion of pain in fibromyalgia, see R. M. Bennett. 'Beyond fibromyalgia: ideas on etiology and treatment.' *J Rheumatol* 19:185–191, 1989; D. J. Clauw and G. P. Chrousos. 'Chronic pain and fatigue syndromes: overlapping clinical and neuroendocrine features and potential pathogenic mechanisms.' *Neuroimmunomodulation* 4:134–53, 1997.

32, 33. S. W. Mitchell. 'The evolution of the rest treatment.' *J Nerv Ment Dis* 31:368–373, 1904. Contains the description of Mitchell's early work on phantom limb syndrome. Dr. Bohr's comments are from Groopman's *The New Yorker* 2000 article, pg. 86.

33–36. For research reports that deal with some of the biological, environmental and genetic aspects of pain mechanisms in fibromyalgia, see I. J. Russell, et al. 'Elevated cerebrospinal fluid levels of substance P in patients with the fibromyalgia syndrome.' *Arthritis Rheum* 37:1593–1601, 1994; S. L. Giovengo, et al. 'Increased concentrations of nerve growth factor in cerebrospinal fluid of patients with fibromyalgia.' *J Rheumatol* 26:1564–69, 1999. Evidence for abnormal central processing of pain in fibromyalgia has been demonstrated by the elevated levels of substance P in the CSF. Substance P is a marker for chronic pain. Nerve growth factor up-regulates substance P and intravenous infusions of nerve growth factor caused muscle pain in fibromyalgia patients. J. M. Mountz, et al. 'Fibromyalgia in women. Abnormalities of regional cerebral blood flow in the thalamus and the caudate nucleus are associated with low pain threshold levels.' *Arthritis Rheum* 38:926–938, 1995; R. Kwiatek, et al. 'Regional cerebral blood flow in fibromyalgia: single photon-emission computed tomography evidence of reduction in the pontine tegmentum and thalami.' *Arthritis and Rheumatism* 43:2823–33, 2000. The imaging studies of the brain have been the most dramatic, demonstrating alterations in blood flow in pain sensitive areas of the brain.

36, 37. For discussion of the role of the autonomic nervous system in chronic pain and anticipatory pain factors, see M. Lekander, et al. 'Social support and immune status during and after chemotherapy for breast cancer.' *Acta Oncolgica* 35:31–7, 1996; M. Lekander, et al. 'Neuroimmune relations in patients with fibromyalgia: a positron emission tomography study.' *Neuroscience Letters*. 282:193–6, 2000.

CHAPTER 4

41, 42. For detailed review of the criteria, epidemiology, and clinical manifestations of CFS, see D. Buchwald, et al. 'Chronic fatigue and the chronic fatigue syndrome: Prevalence in a pacific northwest health care system.' *Ann Intern Med* 123:81–88, 1995; A. Schluederberg, et al. 'Chronic fatigue syndrome research. Definition and medical outcome assessment.' *Ann Intern Med* 117:325–331, 1992; A. L. Komaroff and D. S. Buchwald. 'Chronic fatigue syndrome: an update.' *Annual Review of Medicine* 49:1–13, 1998.

42, 43. Quote from Manningham, from R. Manningham. 'The symptoms, nature and causes, and cure of the febricula, or little fever.' J. Robinson, London, 1750. For excellent review of the overlapping clinical manifestations of CFS and fibromyalgia, see M. A. Demitrack. 'Chronic fatigue syndrome and fibromyalgia.' *Psych Clinics N Amer* 21:671–92, 1998. Beard's quotes on pg. 42 are from his 1869 description of neurasthenia: Beard G. M. 'Neurasthenia, or nervous exhaustion.' *Boston Medical and Surgical Journal* 3:217–21, 1869. An extensive historical analysis of neurasthenia, benign myalgic encephalomyelitis and CFS can be found in E. Shorter. *From Paralysis to Fatigue: A History of Psychosomatic Illness in the Modern Era,* New York: The Free Press, 1992; R. A. Aronowitz. *Making Sense of Illness: Science, Society, and Disease,* Cambridge: Cambridge University Press, 1998; and E. Showalter. *Hystories: Hysterical Epidemics and Modern Media,* New York: Columbia University Press, 1997. These books discuss the controversies of symptoms, syndromes, and diagnostic labels.

43, 44. The initial 1980s reports describing a new CFS epidemic around Lake Tahoe and subsequent search for an infectious etiology are found in S. E. Straus, et al. 'Persisting illness and fatigue in adults with evidence of Epstein-Barr virus infection.' *Ann Intern Med* 102:7–16, 1985 and W. C. Hellinger, et al. 'Chronic fatigue syndrome and the diagnostic utility of antibody to Epstein-Barr virus early antigen.' *JAMA* 260:971–973, 1988. For historical and scientific discussion of a potential infectious etiology of CFS, see M. Sharpe. 'Chronic fatigue syndrome.' *Psychiatric Clin N Amer* 19:549–73, 1996; S. Wessely. 'Old wine in new bottles: neurasthenia and "ME."' *Psychol Med* 20:35–53, 1990; A. L. Komaroff. 'The biology of chronic fatigue syndrome.' *Amer J Med* 108:169–171, 2000; S. Wessely. 'The epidemiology of chronic fatigue syndrome.' *Epidemiol Rev* 17:139–51, 1995; S. Wessely, et al. 'Postinfectious fatigue: prospective cohort study in primary care.'

Lancet 345:1333–1338, 1995.

46. Quote from Wessely on pg. 46 is found in, S. Wessely. 'Chronic fatigue: Symptom and syndrome.' *Ann Intern Med* 134:841, 2001.

47. For more on the cognitive disturbances in CFS and fibromyalgia, see F. Friedberg, et al. 'Symptom patterns in long-duration chronic fatigue syndrome.' *J Psychosom Res* 48:59–68, 2000; V. Michiels, et al. 'Neuropsychological functioning in CFS.' *Acta Psychiat Scand* 103:84–93, 2001; G. M. Grace, et al. 'Concentration and memory deficits in patients with fibromyalgia syndrome.' *J Clin Exp Neuropsychol* 21:477–87, 1999.

47. Quote from H. Johnson. *Osler's Web,* New York: Crown, 1996. Hillary Johnson, a staff reporter for a number of prestigious journals and newspapers, spent nine years investigating CFS. This book makes a dramatic statement that the medical research establishment does not take CFS seriously. Her book raises important questions, but much of the scientific evidence that she presents is biased and her major points have never been validated.

47. To review some important studies of the central nervous system's role in CFS, see A. L. Komaroff. 'The biology of chronic fatigue syndrome.' *Am J Med* 108:169–71, 2000; R. B. Schwartz, et al. 'SPECT imaging of the brain: Comparison of findings in patients with chronic fatigue syndrome, AIDS dementia complex, and major unipolar depression.' *Am J Radiol* 162:943–951, 1994; J. Deluca, et al. 'Neuropsychological impairments in chronic fatigue syndrome, multiple sclerosis, and depression.' *J Neurol Neurosurg Psychiatry* 58:38–43, 1995; M. Sharpe, et al. 'Increased brain serotonin function in men with chronic fatigue syndrome.' *BMJ* 315:164–5, 1997; M. Siobhan, et al. 'Cerebral perfusion in chronic fatigue syndrome and depression.' *Brit J Psych* 176:550–56, 2000.

46–48. Research on neuro-hormonal and immune changes in CFS can be found in M. A. Demitrack and L. J. Crofford. 'Evidence for and pathophysiologic implications of hypothalamic-pituitary-adrenal axis dysregulation in fibromyalgia and chronic fatigue syndrome.' *Ann New York Acad Sci* 840:684–97, 1998; A. J. Cleare, et al. 'Contrasting neuroendocrine responses in depression and chronic fatigue syndrome.' *J Affect Disord* 34:283–89, 1995; A. Kavelaars, et al. 'Disturbed neuroendocrine-immune interactions in chronic-fatigue syndrome.' *J Endocrinology & Metabolism* 85:692–696, 2000; G. Moorkens, et al. 'Characterization of pituitary function with emphasis on GH secretion in the chronic fatigue syndrome.' *Clin*

Endocrinol 53:99–106, 2000; K. De Meirleir, et al. 'A 37 kDa 2-5A binding protein as a potential biochemical marker for chronic fatigue syndrome.' *Amer J Med* 108:99–105, 2000.

48, 49. I. Bou-Holaigah, et al. 'The relationship between neurally mediated hypotension and the chronic fatigue syndrome.' *JAMA* 274:961–967, 1995; P. C. Rowe, et al. 'Fludocortisone acetate to treat neurally mediated hypotension in chronic fatigue syndrome.' *JAMA* 285:52–9, 2001. These papers discuss the autonomic nervous system involvement in CFS. Treatment of orthostatic hypotension was not very effective in CFS.

49. For treatment of CFS, see S. Reid, et al. 'Chronic fatigue syndrome.' *BMJ* 320:292–6, 2000; E. Blondel-Hill and S. D. Shafran. 'Treatment of the chronic fatigue syndrome – a review and practical guide.' *Drugs* 46:639–651, 1993; M. Sharpe, et al. 'Chronic fatigue syndrome. A practical guide to assessment and management.' *Gen Hosp Psychiat* 19:185–99, 1997.

49. For more opinions and reviews about CFS as a specific illness, see S. E. Abbey and P. E. Garfinkel. 'Neurasthenia and chronic fatigue syndrome: the role of culture in the making of a diagnosis.' *Am J Psychiatry* 148:1638–1646, 1991; J. T. Lynn. 'On medical uncertainty.' *Am J Med* 96:186–187, 1994; R. Mayou and M. Sharpe. 'Diagnosis, disease and illness.' *Quarterly J Med* 88:827–31, 1995. For an in-depth discussion that presents the pros and cons regarding the diagnosis of illnesses when no disease is present, see A. Kleinman. *The Illness Narratives: Suffering, Healing and the Human Condition,* Basic Books, 1988. For other controversial discussions of this topic, see the books by Shorter, Showalter and Aronowitz.

50. Quote on pg. 50, from Komaroff, *Amer J Med,* 2000.

CHAPTER 5

53, 54. B. Hedenberg-Magnusson, et al. 'Symptoms and signs of temporomandibular disorders in patients with fibromyalgia and local myalgia of the temporomandibular system. A comparative study.' *Acta Odontologica Scandinavica* 55:344–49, 1997.

55–56. For more information on the relationship of myofascial pain to fibromyalgia, see D. G. Simons and J. G. Travell. 'Myofascial origins of low back pain.' *Postgrad Med* 73:99–99, 1983; D. G. Simons. 'Myofascial pain syndromes: Where are we? Where are we going?' *Arch Phys Med Rehabil*

69:207–212, 1988; A. Okifuji, et al. 'Comparison of generalized and localized hyperalgesia in patients with recurrent headache and fibromyalgia.' *Psychosom Med* 61:771–780, 1999; F. Wolfe, et al. 'The fibromyalgia and myofascial pain syndromes: a preliminary study of tender points and trigger points in persons with fibromyalgia, myofascial pain syndrome and no disease.' *J Rheumatol* 19:944–951, 1992.

56, 57. For review of muscular or tension headaches, see S. D. Siberstein. 'Tension-type headaches.' *Headache* 34:S2–S7, 1994; M. Leone, et al. 'Cervicogenic headache: a critical review of the current diagnostic criteria.' *Pain* 78:1–5, 1998.

57–60. Discussion of headaches, with a focus on the clinical and biological aspects of migraine, see A. Rapoport and J. Edmeads. 'Migraine: the evolution of our knowledge.' *Archives of Neurology* 57:1221–1223, 2000; G. W. Smentana. 'The diagnostic value of historical features in primary headache syndromes: a comprehensive review.' *Arch Intern Med* 160:2729–37, 2000. The quotes found on pp. 58 and 59 are from, O. Sacks. *Migraine: Revised and Expanded*. Berkeley, University of California Press, 1992, pp. 7, 26. This is a beautifully written book about all aspects of migraine. For role of Freud, see A. Karwautz, et al. 'Freud and migraine: the beginning of a psychodynamically oriented view of headache a hundred years ago.' *Cephalalgia* 16:22–26, 1996.

59, 60. The central nervous system changes in migraine and their relationship to brain research reports in fibromyalgia, CFS, and depression are discussed in J. Olesen. 'Understanding the biological basis of migraine.' *N Eng J Med* 331:1713–1714, 1994; T. Paiva, et al. 'The relationship between headaches and sleep disturbances.' *Headache* 35:590–596, 1995; S. K. Aurora and K. M. Welch. 'Migraine: imaging the aura.' *Current Opin in Neurology* 13:273–276, 2000; H. Miranda, et al. 'Depression scores following migraine treatment in patients attending a specialized centre for headache and neurology.' *Headache* 41:680–4, 2001; M. Nicolodi and F. Sicuteri. 'Fibromyalgia and migraine, two faces of the same mechanism. Serotonin as the common clue for pathogenesis and therapy.' *Adv Exp Med Biol* 398:373–79, 1996; M. Nicolodi, et al. 'Changes in the concentrations of amino acids in the cerebrospinal fluid that correlate with pain in patients with fibromyalgia: implications for nitric acid pathways.' *Pain* 87:201–211, 2000. This last report suggests that nitrous oxide pain pathways may be involved in both fibromyalgia and migraine.

60–62. Therapy for migraine and muscular headaches and the overlap with the treatment of fibromyalgia, as well as role of trauma is discussed in, M. Botney and H. L. Fields. 'Amitriptyline potentiates morphine analgesia by a direct action on the central nervous system.' *Ann Neurol* 13:160–64, 1983; R. K. Cady, et al. 'Treatment of acute migraine with subcutaneous sumatriptan.' *JAMA* 265:2831–36, 1991; D. Deleu and Y. Hanssens. 'Current and emerging second-generation triptans in acute migraine therapy: a comparative review.' *J Clin Pharmacol* 40:687–700, 2000. Quote on pp. 61–62, see Sacks, 1990, pg. 124.

CHAPTER 6

67–69. The clinical, diagnostic, and epidemiological aspects of IBS, including the Rome diagnostic criteria, are reviewed in D. A. Drossman. 'Irritable bowel syndrome: a multifactorial disorder.' *Hosp Prac* 95–108, 1988; K. W. Olden and D. A. Drossman. 'Psychologic and psychiatric aspects of gastrointestinal disease.' *Medical Clin North America* 84:1313–1327, 2000; R. D. Rothstein. 'Irritable bowel syndrome.' *Medical Clin North America* 84:1247–1257, 2000; F. Creed, et al. 'Health-related quality of life and health care costs in severe, refractory irritable bowel syndrome.' *Ann Intern Med* 134:860–67, 2001.

68, 69. For studies on similarities and co-occurrence of fibromyalgia and IBS, see A. D. Sperber. 'Fibromyalgia in the irritable bowel syndrome: studies of prevalence and clinical implications.' *Am J Gastro* 94:3541–3546, 1999; L. Chang. 'Differences in somatic perception in female patients with irritable bowel syndrome with and without fibromyalgia.' *Pain* 84:297–307, 2000.

70, 71. For discussion of the pathophysiology of IBS, see J. McLaughlin. 'The brain-gut axis in health and disease.' *Royal College of Physicians* 34:475–477, 2000; J. D. Wood. 'Enteric nervous system, serotonin and the irritable bowel syndrome.' *Current Opinion in Gastroenterology* 17:91–97, 2001; D. A. Drossman. 'Do psychosocial factors define symptom severity and patient status in irritable bowel syndrome?' *Am J Med* 107:41S–50S, 1999; M. Camilleri, et al. 'Visceral hypersensitivity: facts, speculations, and challenges.' *Gut* 48:125–131, 2001. Quote on pg. 70, from Olden, Drossman, 2000.

70, 71. The association of IBS and fibromyalgia with abuse, emotional, and physical trauma is discussed in E. A. Walker, et al. 'Psychosocial factors in fibromyalgia compared with rheumatoid arthritis: II. Sexual, physical, and emotional abuse and neglect.' *Psychosom Med* 59:572–77, 1997; E. A. Walker, et al. 'Adult health status of women with histories of child abuse and neglect.' *Am J Med* 107:332–339, 1999; H. M. Finestone. 'Chronic pain and health care utilization in women with a history of childhood sexual abuse.' *Child Abuse and Neglect* 24:547–556, 2000; M. B. Stein and E. Barrett-Connor. 'Sexual assault and physical health: findings from a population-based study of older adults.' *Psychosom Med* 62: 838–843, 2000; U. M. Anderberg, et al. 'The impact of life events in female patients with fibromyalgia and in female healthy controls.' *European Psychiatry* 15:295–301, 2000; M. G. Newman, et al. 'The relationship of childhood sexual abuse and depression with somatic symptoms and medical utilization.' *Psychological Med* 30:1063–1077, 2000; F. Creed. 'The relationship between psychosocial parameters and outcome in irritable bowel syndrome.' *Am J Med* 107:74S–80S, 1999; J. J. Sherman, et al. 'Prevalence and impact of posttraumatic stress disorder–like symptoms in patients with fibromyalgia syndrome.' *Clin J Pain* 169:127–34, 2000; R. W. Alexander, et al. 'Sexual and physical abuse in women with fibromyalgia: Association with outpatient health care utilization and pain medication usage.' *Arthritis Care Res* 11:102–115, 1998.

71. Teicher's quote on pg. 71 from: Y. Ito, et al. 'Preliminary evidence for aberrant cortical development in abused children.' *J Neuropsych Clin Neurosciences* 10:298–307, 1998. This important study demonstrated that abused children had brain developmental structural alterations. Early life events that are traumatic, such as physical or sexual abuse, may permanently alter the biological response to stress and to pain.

71, 72. Treatment of IBS is reviewed in J. Jailwala, et al. 'Pharmacologic treatment of the irritable bowel syndrome.' *Ann Intern Med* 133:136–147, 2000; M. J. Farthing. 'Irritable bowel syndrome: new pharmaceutical approaches to treatment.' *Bailieres Clin Rheumatol* 13:461–471, 1999; M. Camilleri. 'Therapeutic approach to the patient with irritable bowel syndrome.' *Am J Med* 107:27S–32S, 1999; J. L. Jackson, et al. 'Treatment of functional gastrointestinal disorders with antidepressant medications: a meta-analysis.' *Amer J Med* 108:65–72, 2000.

CHAPTER 7

75. This study is from D. Buskila, et al. 'Increased rates of fibromyalgia follow-ing cervical spine injury. A controlled study of 161 cases of traumatic injury.' *Arthritis Rheum* 40:446–52, 1997.

76–78. The quotes on pg. 76 are from *The Wall Street Journal,* 11 Nov, 1999 and on pg. 77 from a transcript of the 20 March, 2000 *20/20* programme. The study mentioned on pg. 77 was presented at the 2000 American College of Rheumatology national meeting and was titled 'Prevalence of Chiari mal-formation and cervical stenosis in fibromyalgia.' The authors were Daniel Clauw, Robert Bennett, Frank Petzke, and Michael Rosner. Undergoing an extensive neurological examination, a detailed symptom questionnaire, and MRI of the posterior fossa of the brain and the cervical spine were thirty-eight fibromyalgia patients and twenty-three age- and sex-matched controls. The MRIs were interpreted by two radiologists who did not know the diag-nosis. No differences were noted between the fibromyalgia patients and the normal controls in terms of Chiari malformation or cervical stenosis. The neurosurgeon, Dr. Rosner, also evaluated the MRIs without knowledge of the diagnosis and judged that 47 percent of fibromyalgia patients and 50 per-cent of controls were possible surgical candidates. A position statement from the American Association of Neurologic Surgeons stated, 'there is no scien-tific evidence that fibromyalgia and chronic fatigue syndrome are neurolog-ical disorders or that they require surgical intervention.' For greater discussion of the relationship of trauma to fibromyalgia, also see K. P. White. 'Trauma and fibromyalgia.' *Semin Arthritis Rheum* 29:200–16, 2000.

78, 79. For discussion on the status of an infectious etiology for CFS and fibromyalgia, see D. Buchwald, et al. 'A chronic illness characterized by fatigue, neurological and immunologic disorders, and active human her-pesvirus type 6 infection.' *Ann Intern Med* 116:103–113, 1992; D. V. Ablashi, et al. 'Frequent HHV-6 reactivation in multiple sclerosis (MS) and chronic fatigue syndrome (CFS) patients.' *J Clin Virology* 16:179–191, 2000; D. Buchwald, et al. 'Postinfectious chronic fatigue: a distinct syn-drome?' *Clin Infect Dis* 23:385–87, 1996. A. Lindal, et al. 'Anxiety disor-ders: a result of long-term chronic fatigue – the psychiatric characteristics of the sufferers of Iceland disease.' *Acta Neurologica Scand* 96:158–62, 1997; T. Rea, et al. 'A prospective study of tender points and fibromyalgia during and after an acute viral infection.' *Arch Intern Med* 159:865–70, 1999; I. H. Wittrup, et al. 'Comparison of viral antibodies in 2 groups of patients with fibromyalgia.' *J Rheumatol* 28:601–3, 2001. Quote on pg. 79 is from Johnson's *Osler's Web*, pg. 671.

79–83. For discussions of the clinical aspects, diagnostic, and therapeutic guidelines of Lyme disease and its relationship to fibromyalgia and CFS, see E. G. Seltzer, et al. 'Long-term outcomes of persons with Lyme disease.' *JAMA* 283:5:609–616, 2000; L. H. Sigal. 'The Lyme disease controversy. Social and financial costs of misdiagnosis and mismanagement.' *Arch Intern Med* 156:1493–1500, 1996; P. Tugwell, et al. 'Laboratory evaluation in the diagnosis of Lyme disease.' *Ann Intern Med* 127:1109–23, 1997; G. Nichol, et al. 'Test-treatment strategies for patients suspected of having Lyme disease: A cost-effectiveness analysis.' *Ann Intern Med* 128:37–48, 1998; V. M. Hsu, et al. ' 'Chronic Lyme disease' as the incorrect diagnosis in patients with fibromyalgia.' *Arthritis Rheum* 36:1493–1500, 1993; M. S. Klempner, et al. 'Two controlled trials of antibiotic treatment in patients with persistent symptoms and a history of Lyme disease.' *N Eng J Med* 345:85–92, 2001; A. C. Steere. 'Medical progress: Lyme disease.' *N Engl J Med* 345:115–125, 2001. The quotes on pp. 82–83 are from the 8 July, 2000 *New York Times* article by David Grann, 'Stalking Doctor Steere,' pp. 56–7.

83, 84. Discussions of multiple chemical sensitivities are found in, C. M. Brodsky. '"Allergic to everything": a medical subculture.' *Psychosomatics* 24:731–42, 1983; G. E. Simon, et al. 'Immunologic, psychological, and neuropsychological factors in multiple chemical sensitivity. A controlled study.' *Ann Intern Med* 119:97–103, 1993; G. E. Simon, et al. 'Allergic to life: psychological factors in environmental illness.' *Am J Psychiatry* 147:901–6, 1990; D. W. Black, et al. 'Environmental illness: a controlled study of 26 subjects with '20th century disease.' ' *JAMA* 264:3166–3170, 1990; A. C. Chester and P. H. Levine. 'Concurrent sick building syndrome and chronic fatigue syndrome: epidemic neuromyasthenia revisited.' *Clin Infect Dis* 18:S43–S48, 1994.

CHAPTER 8

90, 91. M. S. Micale. *Approaching Hysteria: Disease and Its Interpretations,* Princeton: Princeton University Press, 1995. This book provides a detailed discussion of hysteria from a medical and cultural viewpoint. The quote about hysteria from Plato is on pg. 18 of this book.

91–93. Willis quote on pg. 91 from Willis, T: *An essay of the pathology of the Brain and Nervous Shock in which Convulsive Diseases are Treated of.* Dring, Leigh and Harper, 1684. For a comprehensive review of symptoms commonly seen in primary care practice that are not related to a known disease, see the supplement issue of the *Ann Intern Med,* 134:801–926, 2001. Other reviews of functional syndromes and unexplained somatic illnesses, see G. E. Simon, et al. 'An international study of the relation between somatic symptoms and depression.' *N Engl J Med* 341:1329–35, 1999; R. Mayou and M. Sharpe. 'Diagnosis, disease and illness.' *Quarterly J Med* 88:827–31, 1995; M. Sharpe. 'Chronic fatigue syndrome.' *Psychiatric Clin N Amer* 19:549–73, 1996; S. Kisely, et al. 'A comparison between somatic symptoms with and without clear organic cause: results of an international study.' *Psychol Med* 27:1011–9, 1997; A. J. Barsky and J. F. Borus. 'Functional somatic syndromes.' *Ann Intern Med* 130:910–21, 1999.

93. Two books by Drs. Barsky and Shorter, both psychiatrists, provide an interesting, albeit psychologically oriented, look at symptoms that cannot be explained by organic disease: A. J. Barsky. *Worried Sick: Our Troubled Quest for Wellness,* Boston: Little, Brown, 1998; E. Shorter. *From Paralysis to Fatigue: A History of Psychosomatic Illness in the Modern Era,* New York: The Free Press, 1992, which includes the quote from Shorter found on pg. 10 of his book.

93, 94. J. E. Sarno. *The Mindbody Prescription: Healing the Body, Healing the Pain,* New York: Warner Books, 1998. Sarno's book addresses what, according to him, are physical disorders caused by repressed, unconscious feelings. The quote on pg. 94 is found on pg. 50 of his book. For further discussion of the overlap of somatization with pain disorders, see S. Benjamin, et al. 'The association between chronic widespread pain and mental disorder.' *Arthritis Rheum* 43:561–7, 2000 and J. McBeth, et al. 'Features of somatization predict the onset of widespread pain.' *Arthritis Rheum* 44:940–6, 2001.

94–95. Barsky's quote is from Groopman's *The New Yorker* article, pg. 86.

95. For a review of the interactions of genetic and environmental factors in pain processing: N. A. Gillespie, et al. 'The genetic aetiology of somatic distress.' *Psychological Medicine* 30:1051–1061, 2000; A. J. Barsky, et al. 'Somatic symptom reporting in women and men.' *J Gen Intern Med* 16:266–75, 2001.

CHAPTER 9

100, 101. The classification criteria of depression is from: American Psychiatric Association. *Diagnostic and Statistical Manual of Mental Disorders*, American Psychiatric Association: Washington, D.C., 1994.

100–102. For general discussions about depression and medical illness, see A. Rozanski, et al. 'Impact of psychological factors on the pathogenesis of cardiovascular disease and implications for therapy.' *Circulation* 99:212–217, 1999; T. P. Guck, et al. 'Assessment and treatment of depression following myocardial infarction.' *Amer Family Physician* 64:641–8, 2001; D. E. Bush, et al. 'Even minimal symptoms of depression increase mortality risk after acute myocardial infarction.' *Amer J Cardiol* 88:337–41, 2001; J. L. Januzzi Jr., et al. 'The influence of anxiety and depression on outcomes of patients with coronary artery disease.' *Arch Intern Med* 60:1913–21, 2000; 'Treating depression and anxiety in primary care.' *N Eng J Med* 326:1080–1084, 1992; J. Angst and K. Merikangas. 'The depressive spectrum: diagnostic classification and course.' *J Affect Disord* 45:31–9, 1997. For a sobering book about depression and suicide, see K. R. Jamison. *Night Falls Fast: Understanding Suicide,* New York: Alfred A. Knopf, 1999.

101, 102. For reviews of the associations of mood disturbances with fibromyalgia and related functional syndromes, see D. L. Goldenberg. 'Psychiatric and psychological aspects of fibromyalgia syndrome.' *Rheum Dis Clin N Am* 15:105–114, 1989; A. J. Gruber, J. I. Hudson, and H. G. Pope Jr. 'The management of treatment-resistant depression in disorders on the interface of psychiatry and medicine.' *Psychiatric Clin N Amer* 19:351–69, 1996; J. I. Hudson, et al. 'Comorbidity of fibromyalgia with medical and psychiatric disorders.' *Am J Med* 92:363–367, 1992; J. McBeth and A. J. Silman. 'The role of psychiatric disorders in fibromyalgia.' *Curr Rheumatol Rep* 3:157–64, 2001; S. A. Epstein, et al. 'Psychiatric disorders in patients with fibromyalgia.' *Psychosomatics* 40:57–63, 1999.

100–101. An excellent book on sleep is P. Hauri and S. Linde. *No More Sleepless Nights,* New York: John Wiley and Sons, 1990.

102. The quote is from W. Styron. *Darkness Visible,* New York: Vintage Books, 1992, pg. 34.

101–104. Some books that tackle different facets of depression, including the historical, see A. Kleinman. *The Illness Narratives: Suffering, Healing and the Human Condition,* Basic Books, 1988; K. R. Jamison. *An Unquiet Mind: A Memoir of Moods and Madness,* New York: Vintage Books, 1995; E. Shorter. *A History of Psychiatry,* New York: John Wiley & Sons, Inc., 1997. For a thought-provoking editorial on the organic versus functional dichotomy in neurology and psychiatry, see B. H. Price, et al. 'Neurology and psychiatry: closing the great divide.' *Neurology* 54:8–14, 2000.

104–106. For more studies on the relationship of neurohormones, immunity, and the autonomic nervous system in fibromyalgia, depression, and related illnesses, see K. J. Ressler et al. 'Role of serotonergic and noradrenergic systems in the pathophysiology of depression and anxiety disorders.' *Depression & Anxiety.* 12 *Suppl* 1:2–19, 2000; J. W. Kasckow, et al. 'Corticotropin-releasing hormone in depression and post-traumatic stress disorder.' *Peptides.* 22:845–51, 2001: B. H. Natelson, et al. 'Is depression associated with immune activation?' *J Affective Disord* 53:179–84, 1999; J. Albrecht, et al. 'A controlled study of cellular immune function in affective disorders before and during somatic therapy.' *Psychiatr Res* 15:185–193, 1985; L. Bradley, et al. 'Sertraline Hydrochloride (sertraline (Lustral)) alters pain threshold, sensory discrimination ability, and functional brain activity in patients with fibromyalgia (FM): A randomized controlled trial (RCT).' *Arthritis Rheum* 41:259, 1998; D. J. Torpy, et al. 'Responses of the sympathetic nervous system and the hypothalamic-pituitary-adrenal axis to interleukin-6: A pilot study in fibromyalgia.' *Arthritis Rheum* 43:872–880, 2000; I. Bou-Holaigah, et al. 'Provocation of hypotension and pain during upright tilt table testing in adults with fibromyalgia.' *Clinical & Experimental Rheumatology* 15:239–46, 1997; M. J. Schwarz, et al. 'Relationship of substance P, 5-hydroxyindole acetic acid and tryptophan in serum of fibromyalgia patients.' *Neurosci Lett* 259:196–98, 1999.

106, 107. Studies on the impact of mood on the prognosis and outcome in fibromyalgia include: J. I. Hudson and H. G. Pope. 'The concept of affective spectrum disorder: Relationship to fibromyalgia and other syndromes of chronic fatigue and chronic muscle pain.' *Baillieres Clin Rheumatol* 8:839–856, 1994; D. L. Goldenberg, et al. 'A model to assess severity and impact of fibromyalgia.' *J Rheumatol* 22:2313–18, 1995; G. Granges, et al; 'Fibromyalgia syndrome: assessment of the severity of the condition 2 years after diagnosis.' *J Rheumatol* 21:523–529, 1994; L. A. Aaron, et al. 'Psychiatric diagnoses in patients with fibromyalgia are related to health care-seeking behavior rather than to illness.' *Arthritis Rheum* 39:436–445, 1996.

107, 108. For an in-depth review of antidepressants and their role in fibromyalgia and chronic pain, see D. L. Goldenberg, et al. 'A randomized, double-blind crossover trial of fluoxetine and amitriptyline in the treatment of fibromyalgia.' *Arthritis Rheum* 39:1852–59, 1996; A. J. Gruber, et al. 'The management of treatment-resistant depression in disorders on the interface of psychiatry and medicine.' *Psychiatric Clin N Amer* 19:351–69, 1996; G. S. Alarcon and L. A. Bradley. 'Advances in the treatment of fibromyalgia: current status and future directions.' *Am J Med Sci* 315:397–404, 1998.

107–109. General discussions of pharmacological and non-pharmacological treatment of depression are found in: M. B. Keller, et al. 'Maintenance phase efficacy of sertraline for chronic depression.' *JAMA* 280:1665–1672, 1998; J. Mendlewicz. 'Optimising antidepressant use in clinical practice: towards criteria for antidepressant selection.' *Brit J Psych* 42:S1–3, 2001; J. E. Barrett, et al. 'The treatment effectiveness project. A comparison of the effectiveness of paroxetine, problem-solving therapy, and placebo in the treatment of minor depression and dysthymia in primary care patients: background and research plan.' *Gen Hospital Psych* 21:260–73, 1999; C. D. Mulrow, et al. 'Efficacy of newer medications for treating depression in primary care patients.' *Amer J Med* 108:54–64, 2000; E. Richelson. 'Pharmacology of antidepressants.' *Mayo Clin Proc* 76:511–27, 2001; S. M. Cheer, et al. 'Fluoxetine: a review of its therapeutic potential in the treatment of depression associated with physical illness.' *Drugs* 61:81–110, 2001.

CHAPTER 10

112–114. Two books by Eddington and Wheelwright take very different views of the medical and social factors involved in the Gulf War syndrome: Wheelwright J. *The Irritable Heart*. W. W. Norton & Co. 2001 and Eddington P. *Gassed in the Gulf*. Insignia. 1997. Wheelwright explores Gulf War syndrome from a historical and medical view and notes its overlap with fibromyalgia and CFS. Quote on pg. 112 from Eddington's book, pg. 4 and on pg. 113 from Wheelwright's book, pg. 39. For complete reviews of the Gulf War syndrome, see G. W. Beebe. 'Follow-up studies of World War II and Korean War prisoners. II. Morbidity, disability, and maladjustments.' *Am J Epidemiol* 101:400–22, 1975; R. W. Haley, et al. 'Is there a Gulf War Syndrome? Searching for syndromes by factor analysis of symptoms.' *JAMA* 277:215–22, 1997; A. A. Amato, et al. 'Evaluation of neuromuscular symptoms in veterans of the Persian Gulf War.' *Neurology* 48:4–12, 1997; K. Fukuda, et al. 'Chronic multi-symptom illness affecting air force veterans of the gulf war.' *JAMA* 280:981–988, 1998; C. Unwin, et al. 'Health of UK servicemen who served in Persian Gulf War.' *Lancet* 353:168–178, 1999.

115. Wessely's quote is from Jane Brody's personal health article in *The New York Times,* 16 March, 1999.

115. Joseph's quote is from a transcript of the PBS *Frontline* programme, *Last Battle of the Gulf War,* which was broadcast on PBS on 20 January, 1998.

115–117. The role of stress, see H. Selye. 'The general adaptation syndrome and diseases of adaptation.' *J Clin Endocrinol* 6:217–21, 1946. This is Selye's landmark study on stress. Includes quote on pg. 116. For more recent general research on stress, see P. W. Gold, et al. 'Clinical and biochemical manifestations of depression. Relation to the neurobiology of stress.' *N Eng J Med* 319:348–352, 1988; B. S. McEwen. 'Protective and damaging effects of stress mediators.' *N Eng J Med* 338:171–79, 1998; L. M. Slimmer, et al. 'Stress, medical illness, and depression.' *Semin Clin Neuropsychiatry* 6:12–26, 2001; G. P. Chrousos and P. W. Gold. 'The concepts of stress and stress system disorders: Overview of physical and behavioral homeostasis.' *JAMA* 267:1244–52, 1992.

117. Key reports of the effect of stress on immune function include: L. E. Cluff. 'Asian influenza: infection, disease and psychological factors.' *Arch Intern Med* 117:159–163, 1966; S. Cohen, et al. 'Psychological stress and susceptibility to the common cold.' *N Eng J Med* 325:606–612, 1991; W. B. Malarkey, et al. 'The influence of academic stress and season on 24-hour concentrations of growth hormone and prolactin.' *J Clin Endocrinol Metab* 73:1089–1092, 1991.

117, 118. Ader's breakthrough research leading to the science of psycho-neuroimmunology is described in R. Ader and N. Cohen. 'Behaviorally conditioned immunosuppression and murine systemic lupus erythematosus.' *Science* 214:1534–1536, 1982. Mice were conditioned to improve their immune function in an animal model of lupus. For in-depth review of the field of psycho-neuroimmunology, see R. Ader, et al. 'Psychoneuroimmunology: interactions between the nervous system and the immune system.' *Lancet* 345:99–103, 1995. Also see S. Lutgendorf, et al. 'Effects of relaxation and stress on the capsaicin-induced local inflammatory response.' *Psychosom Med* 62:524–534, 2000.

118, 119. Comprehensive books about modifying the stress response for optimal health include: H. Benson. *The Relaxation Response,* New York: Morrow, 1975. J. K. Zinn. *Full Catastrophe Living: Using Wisdom of Your Body and Mind to Face Stress, Pain, and Illness,* New York: Delta, 1990.

119. For more on relaxation techniques and cognitive behavioural treatment of fibromyalgia and CFS, see D. L. Goldenberg, et al. 'A controlled study of a stress-reduction, cognitive-behavioral treatment programme in fibromyalgia.' *J Musculoskeletal Pain* 2:53–66, 1994; 'NIH Technology assessment panel on integration of behavioral and relaxation approaches into the treatment of chronic pain and insomnia.' *JAMA* 276:313–18, 1996; A. Deale, et al. 'Cognitive behavior therapy for chronic fatigue syndrome.' *Am J Psychiatry* 154:408–14, 1997. Quote on pg. 118, see Selye, 1946.

CHAPTER 11

121–123. For a comprehensive book reviewing the history, mechanisms, and treatments of chronic pain, see S. Fishman and L. Berger. *The War on Pain,* New York: HarperCollins Publishers, 2000. Also see R. K. Portenoy. 'Current pharmacotherapy of chronic pain.' *Journal of Pain & Symptom Management* 19:S16–S20, 2000.

123–127. Clinical trials of analgesics, antidepressants, and other drugs in fibromyalgia, see L. J. Leventhal. 'Management of fibromyalgia.' *Ann Intern Med* 131:850–8, 1999; G. S. Carette. 'Chronic pain syndromes.' *Ann Rheum Dis* 55:497–501, 1996; D. L. Goldenberg. 'Management of fibromyalgia syndrome.' *Rheum Dis Clin N Am* 15:499–512, 1989; R. G. Godfrey. 'A guide to the understanding and use of tricyclic antidepressants in the overall management of fibromyalgia and other chronic pain syndromes.' *Arch Intern Med* 156:1047–52, 1996; P. Hannonen, et al. 'A randomized, double-blind, placebo-controlled study of moclobemide and amitriptyline in the treatment of fibromyalgia in females without psychiatric disorder.' *Brit J Rheumatol* 37:1279–86, 1998; M. L. Chambliss. 'Are serotonin uptake inhibitors useful in chronic pain syndromes such as fibromyalgia or diabetic neuropathy.' *Arch Fam Medicine* 7:470–1, 1998

G. Biasi, et al. 'Tramadol in the fibromyalgia syndrome: a controlled clinical trial versus placebo.' *Int J Clin Pharmacol Res* 18:13–19, 1998; J. H. Juhl. 'Fibromyalgia and the serotonin pathway.' *Altern Med* 3:36775, 1998; L. A. Rossy, et al. 'A meta-analysis of fibromyalgia treatment interventions.' *Ann Behavioral Med* 21:180–91, 1999.

126, 127. Medications for sleep disturbances are discussed in W. J. Reynolds, et al. 'The effects of cyclobenzaprine on sleep physiology and symptoms in patients with fibromyalgia.' *J Rheumatol* 18:452–454, 1991; J. Montplaisir, et al. 'Clinical, polysomnographic, and genetic characteristics of restless legs syndrome: a study of 133 patients diagnosed with new standard criteria.' *Movement Disorder* 12:61–65, 1997; H. Moldofsky, et al. 'The effect of Zolpidem in patients with fibromyalgia: A dose ranging, double-blind, placebo controlled, modified crossover study.' *J Rheumatol* 23:529–533, 1996; S. L. Bartusch, et al. 'Clonazepam for the treatment of lancinating phantom limb pain.' *Clin J Pain* 12:59–62, 1996.

128. The popular book that proposes treating fibromyalgia with guaifenesin is R. P. Amand and C. C. Marek. *What Your Doctor May Not Tell You About Fibromyalgia,* New York: Warner Books, 1999. Other nontraditional and alternative remedies for fibromyalgia are discussed in I. J. Russell, et al. 'Treatment of fibromyalgia syndrome with super malic.' *J Rheumatol* 22:953–8, 1995; G. Citera, et al. 'The effect of melatonin in patients with primary fibromyalgia. A pilot study.' *Arthritis Rheum* 40:S43, 1997; S. Ozgocmen, et al. 'Effect of omega-3 fatty acids in the management of fibromyalgia syndrome.' *Inter J Clin Pharmacol Therap* 38:362–3, 2000; K. Kaartinen, et al. 'Vegan diet alleviates fibromyalgia symptoms.' *Scand J Rheumatology* 29:308–13, 2000; B. Bramwell, et al. 'The use of ascorbigen in the treatment of fibromyalgia patients: a preliminary trial.' *Alternative Med Review* 5:455–62, 2000

128–129. New medications being tested in fibromyalgia, see U. Haus, et al. 'Oral treatment of fibromyalgia with tropisetron given over 28 days: influence on functional and vegatative symptoms, psychometric parameters and pain.' *Scand J Rheumatol* 29:55–58, 2000; W. Muller and T. Stratz. 'Results of the intravenous administration of tropisetron in fibromyalgia patients.' *Scand J Rheumatol* 29:59–65, 2000; M. B. Scharf, et al. 'Effect of gamma-hydroxybutyrate on pain, fatigue, and the alpha sleep anomaly in patients with fibromyalgia.' *J Rheumatol* 25:1986–90, 1998; T. C. Birdsall. '5-Hydroxytryptophan: a clinically-effective serotonin precursor.' *Alternat Med Review* 3:271–80, 1998; I. J. Russell, et al. 'Lymphocyte markers and natural killer cell activity in fibromyalgia syndrome: effects of low-dose, sublingual use of human interferon-alpha.' *J Interferon & Cytokine Res* 19:969–78, 1999; T. Graven-Nielsen, et al. 'Ketamine reduces muscle pain, temporal summation, and referred pain in fibromyalgia patients.' *Pain* 85:483–91, 2000; G. Citera, et al. 'The effect of melatonin in patients with fibromyalgia: a pilot study.' *Clin Rheumatology* 19:9–13, 2000.

CHAPTER 12

131–133. Review of chiropractic care in general medical disorders, see J. Balon, et al. 'A comparison of active and simulated chiropractic manipulation as adjunctive treatment for childhood asthma.' *N Eng J Med* 339:1013–20, 1998; G. B. J. Andersson, et al. 'A comparison of osteopathic spinal manipulation with standard care for patients with low back pain.' *N Eng J Med* 341:1426–1431, 1999. Chiropractic and manipulative treatment for fibromyalgia and other musculoskeletal pain disorders is discussed in G. Hains and F. Hains. 'A combined ischemic compression and spinal manipulation in the treatment of fibromyalgia: a preliminary estimate of dose efficacy.' *J Manip Physiological Therap* 23:225–230, 2000; J. J. Fiechtner and R. R. Brodeur. 'Manual and manipulation techniques for rheumatic disease.' *Rheum Dis Clin N Am* 26:83–96, 2000.

133, 134. Physical therapy in fibromyalgia, see M. Offenbacher and G. Stucki. 'Physical therapy in the treatment of fibromyalgia.' *Scand J Rheumatol* 29:78–85, 2000.

135, 136. Review of acupuncture in the treatment of fibromyalgia and other pain disorders, see B. M. Berman, et al. 'Is acupuncture effective in the treatment of fibromyalgia?' *J Fam Prac* 48:213–18, 1999; B. M. Berman, et al. 'The evidence for acupuncture as a treatment for rheumatologic conditions.' *Rheum Dis Clin N Am* 26:103–115, 2000; M. T. Wu, et al. 'Central nervous pathway for acupuntcure stimulation: localization of processing with functional MR imaging of the brain-preliminary experience.' *Radiology* 212:133–141, 2001. In the report by Wu, acupuncture's effect on the brain was detected by functional MR imaging. The acupuncture activated the descending antinociceptive pathway and deactivated a number of pain areas in the limbic system of the brain.

136, 137. General discussions of cardiovascular exercise, see M. Pratt. 'Benefits of lifestyle activity vs structured exercise.' *JAMA* 28:375–375, 1999; P. Salmon. 'Effects of physical exercise on anxiety, depression, and sensitivity to stress: a unifying theory.' *Clin Psychol Review* 21:33–61, 2001; M. Babyak, et al. 'Exercise treatment for major depression.' *Psychosomatic Med* 62:633–638, 2000; U. M. Kujala. 'Leisure physical activity and various pain symptoms among adolescents.' *Brit J Sports Medicine* 33:325–328, 1999; P. A. Ades, et al. 'Weight training improves walking endurance in healthy persons.' *Ann Intern Med* 124:568–572, 1996.

137–139. Role of exercise in fibromyalgia, see G. A. McCain. 'Non-medicinal treatments in primary fibromyalgia.' *Rheum Dis Clin N Am* 15:73–90, 1989; C. S. Burckhardt, et al. 'Use of the modified Balke treadmill protocol for determining the aerobic capacity of women with fibromyalgia.' *Arthritis Care Res* 2:165–167, 1989; R. Isomeri, et al. 'Effects of amitriptyline and cardiovascular fitness training on pain in patients with primary fibromyalgia.' *J Musculoskeletal Pain* 1:253–260, 1993; S. E. Gowans, et al. 'A randomized controlled trial of exercise and education for individuals with fibromyalgia.' *Arthritis Care Res* 12:120–28, 1999; C. Ramsey, et al. 'An observer-blinded comparison of supervised and unsupervised aerobic exercise regimens in fibromyalgia.' *Rheumatology* 39:501–505, 2000; G. Granges and G. O. Littlejohn. 'A comparative study of clinical signs in fibromyalgia/fibrositis syndrome, healthy and exercising subjects.' *J Rheumatol* 20:344–351, 1993; A. Häkkinen, et al. 'Strength training induced adaptions in neuromuscular function of premenopausal women with fibromyalgia: comparison with healthy women.' *Ann Rheum Dis* 60:21–26, 2001.

137–139. The role of relaxation techniques, including yoga and meditation, in fibromyalgia and other rheumatic disorders is discussed in S. P. Buckelew, et al. 'Biofeedback/relaxation training and exercise interventions for fibromyalgia: A prospective trial.' *Arthritis Care Res* 11:196–209, 1998; J. Kabat-Zinn. 'An outpatient programme in behavioral medicine for chronic pain patients based on the practice of mindfulness meditation: theoretical considerations and preliminary results.' *Gen Hosp Psychiat* 4:33–47, 1982; K. H. Kaplan, et al. 'The impact of a meditation-based stress reduction programme on fibromyalgia.' *Gen Hosp Psychiat* 15:284–289, 1993; M. Garfinkel and H. R. Schmacher Jr. 'Yoga.' *Rheum Dis Clin N Am* 26:125–132, 2000; J. E. Broderick. 'Mind-body medicine in rheumatologic disease.' *Rheum Dis Clin N Am* 26:161–176, 2000.

137, 138. Role of exercise in CFS, P. Powell, et al. 'Randomized controlled trial of patient education to encourage graded exercise in chronic fatigue syndrome.' *Brit Med J* 322:387–89, 2001. This report demonstrated that outcome and compliance with exercise was much better when CFS patients were given an explanation of the physiological effects of exercise that might reduce CFS symptoms; Also see P. De Becker, et al. 'Exercise capacity in chronic fatigue syndrome.' *Arch Intern Med* 160:3270–3277, 2000. Contains quote from page 136.

138–140. Education programmes in fibromyalgia, see C. S. Burckhardt and A. Bjelle. 'Education programmes for fibromyalgia patients: Description and evaluation.' *Baillieres Clin Rheumatol* 8:935–955, 1994; C. S. Burckhardt, et al. 'A randomized, controlled clinical trial of education and physical training for women with fibromyalgia.' *J Rheumatol* 21:714–720, 1994; O. Kogstad, et al. 'Pain school. Therapeutic offers to patients with fibromyalgia and other non-malignant pain problems.' *Tidsskr Nor Laegeforen* 111:1725–1728, 1991; D. C. Turk, et al. 'Interdisciplinary treatment for fibromyalgia syndrome: Clinical and statistical significance.' *Arthritis Care Res* 11:186–95, 1998.

139, 140. D. E. Yocum, et al. 'Exercise, education, and behavioral modification as alternative therapy for pain and stress in rheumatic disease.' *Rheum Dis Clin N Amer* 26:146–59, 2000. Describes research at the Canyon Ranch Spa in Arizona that documented hormonal, biological, and psychological improvement when arthritis patients participated in a one week intensive programme involving education, stress-reduction techniques, and exercise.

CHAPTER 13

142. For estimates about the use of complementary therapy, see M. Pioro-Boisset, et al. 'Alternative medicine use in fibromyalgia syndrome.' *Arthritis Care Res* 9:13–17, 1996; D. M. Eisenberg, et al. 'Unconventional medicine in the United States. Prevalence, costs, and patterns in use.' *N Eng J Med* 328:246–252, 1993; D. Eisenberg. 'Alternative medical therapies for rheumatologic disorders.' *Arthritis Care Res* 9:1–4, 1996; For general discussions of alternative medicine, see T. J. Kaptchuk and D. M. Eisenberg. 'The persuasive appeal of alternative medicine.' *Ann Intern Med* 129:1061–1066, 1998; C. Ramos-Remus, et al. 'Epidemiology of complementary and alternative practices in rheumatology.' *Rheum Dis Clin N Am* 25:789–804, 1999.

143–144. For review of diet and nutritional therapies in rheumatic illnesses, see C. J. Henderson and R. S. Panush. 'Diets, dietary supplements, and nutritional therapies in rheumatic diseases.' *Rheum Dis Clin N Am* 25:937–968, 1999. Includes quote from Hippocrates on pg. 142.

144–146. Herbal therapy and potential medicinal effects, see L. C. Winslow and D. J. Kroll. 'Herbs as medicines.' *Arch Intern Med* 158:2192–2199, 1998; N. H. Mashour, et al. 'Herbal medicine for the treatment of cardiovascular disease: clinical considerations.' *Arch Intern Med* 158:2225–2234, 1998. For discussion of St. John's wort, see B. Gaster and J. Holroyd. 'St.-John's-wort for depression.' *Arch Intern Med* 160:152–156, 2000. Echinacea, see W. Grimm and H. H. Müller. 'A randomized controlled trial of the effect of fluid extract of *Echinecea purpurea* on the incidence and severity of colds and respiratory infections.' *Amer J Med* 106:138–143, 1999.

145, 146. Examples of adverse reactions to natural or herbal products include: G. M. Woolf, et al. 'Acute hepatitis associated with the Chinese herbal product jin bu huan.' *Ann Intern Med* 121:729–735, 1994; J. L. Vanherweghem, et al. 'Rapidly progressive interstitial renal fibrosis in young women: association with slimming regimen including chinese herbs.' *Lancet* 341:387–391, 1993.

147. Discussion of potential effects and controversy of using magnets to treat medical conditions, see E. Collacott, et al. 'Bipolar permanent magnets for the treatment of chronic low back pain.' *JAMA* 283:1322–1325, 2000; D. H. Trock. 'Electromagnetic fields and magnets: investigational treatment for musculoskeletal disorders.' *Rheum Dis Clin N Am* 26:51–62, 2000.

147, 148. For a review of the history of homeopathy, see A. Weil. *Health and Healing,* Boston: Houghton Mifflin Company, 1995. For articles on homeopathic treatment for fibromyalgia and other rheumatic diseases, see P. Fisher, et al. 'Effect of homeopathic treatment on fibrositis (primary fibromyalgia).' *BMJ* 299:365–366, 1989; L. E. Andrade, et al. 'A randomized controlled trial to evaluate the effectiveness of homeopathy in rheumatoid arthritis.' *Scand J Rheumatol* 20:204–208, 1991; W. B. Jonas, et al.

'Homeopathy and rheumatic disease.' *Rheum Dis Clin N Am* 26:117–123, 2000.

148, 149. Use of complementary therapy in medical conditions and influence of psychological status, see H. J. Burstein, et al. 'Use of alternative medicine by women with early-stage breast cancer.' *N Eng J Med* 340:1733–39, 1999; J. C. Holland. 'Use of alternative medicine – A marker for distress?' *N Eng J Med* 340:1758–59, 1999; P. M. Nicassio, et al. 'Psychosocial factors associated with complementary treatment use in fibromyalgia.' *J Rheumatol* 24:2008–13, 1997. Poor clinical status was associated with use of complementary treatments in fibromyalgia.

150. For two detailed and fascinating books that focus on the placebo effect in medicine, see H. Spiro. *The Power of Hope: A Doctor's Perspective,* New Haven: Yale University Press, 1998 and A. K. Shapiro and E. Shapiro. *The Powerful Placebo: From Ancient Priest to Modern Physician,* Baltimore: The Johns Hopkins University Press, 1997. A. Hrobjartsson, et al. 'Is the placebo powerless?' *N Engl J Med* 344:1594–1602, 2001; J. C. Bailar III. 'The powerful placebo and the Wizard of Oz.' *N Engl J Med* 344:1630–1632, 2001. These recent articles question the power of placebos in clinical trials.

150. Overview of quackery in medicine, see W. T. Jarvis. 'Quackery: the national council against health fraud perspective.' *Rheum Dis Clin N Am* 25:805–814, 1999. Contains quote by Holmes on pg. 150.

151. Various views are taken regarding the use of complementary medicine in the following articles: A. H. Neims. 'Why I would recommend complementary or alternative therapies: a physician's perspective.' *Rheum Dis Clin N Am* 25:845–853, 1999; H. M. Spiro. 'Hope helps: placebos and alternative medicine in rheumatology.' *Rheum Dis Clin N Am* 25:855–887, 1999; J. K. Rao, et al. 'Use of complementary therapies for arthritis among patients of rheumatologists.' *Ann Intern Med* 131: 409–416, 1999; M. Kanning. 'Why I would want to use complementary and alternative therapy: a patient's perspective.' *Rheum Dis Clin N Am* 25:823–831, 1999; N. Kramer. 'Why I would not recommend complementary or alternative therapies: a physician's perspective.' *Rheum Dis Clin N Am* 25:833–843, 1999. Quote from Osler on pg. 151 from A. K. Shapiro and E. Shapiro. *The Powerful Placebo,* pg. 3.

CHAPTER 14

155–158. For general discussions of health information on the Internet, see Gina Kolata, *Web research transforms visit to the doctor. The New York Times* March 6, 2000; Quote on pg. 154 from A. R. Jadad and A. Gagliardi. 'Rating health information on the Internet: navigating to knowledge or to Babel?' *JAMA* 279:611–14, 1998; A. A. Skolnick. 'WHO considers regulating ads, sale of medical products on Internet.' *JAMA* 278:1723–24, 1997; F. A. Sonnenberg. 'Health information on the Internet. Opportunities and pitfalls.' *Arch Intern Med* 157:151–52, 1997; R. Kiley. 'Consumer health information on the Internet.' *J Royal Soc Med* 91:202–3, 1998.

157. Quote from jacket cover, Johnson, *Osler's Web*.

158. See transcript from the 4 Jan, 2000 *Dateline* programme.

158–161. Quotes from Joseph, Rather, and Hale, see transcript of the PBS *Frontline* programme, *Last Battle of the Gulf War,* which was broadcast on PBS on 20 January, 1998.

161. For general discussion of the impact of the media on medical information, see R. A. Aronowitz. *Making Sense of Illness: Science, Society, and Disease,* Cambridge: Cambridge University Press, 1998; D. Nelson. *Selling Silence Revised Edition: How the Press Covers Science and Technology,* New York: W. H. Freeman and Company, 1995; E. W. Campion. 'Power lines, cancer, and fear.' *N Eng J Med* 337:44–46, 1997; M. Angell and J. P. Kassirer. 'Clinical research – what should the public believe?' *N Eng J Med* 331:189–190, 1994.

161, 162. D. L. Goldenberg, A. M. Miller. 'Fibromyalgia on the Internet: A misinformation superhighway.' *Arthritis Rheum* 42:S151, 1999

CHAPTER 15

165, 166. Reviews of doctor-patient relationships and physician reinforcement of illness behaviour. R. M. Glass. 'The patient-physician relationship.' *JAMA* 275:147–48, 1996; D. W. Black. 'Iatrogenic (physician-induced) hypochondriasis.' *Psychosomatics* 37:390–5, 1996.

167–168. For discussion of injuries, the workplace, compensation, and disability in fibromyalgia and related pain disorders, see R. M. Bennett. 'Fibromyalgia and the disability dilemma. A new era in understanding a complex, multidimensional pain syndrome.' *Arthritis Rheum* 39:1627–34, 1996; R. M. Bennett. 'Disabling fibromyalgia: appearance versus reality.' *J*

Rheumatol 20:1820–1824, 1993; K. Capen. 'The courts, expert witnesses and fibromyalgia.' *Can Med Assoc J* 153:206–208, 1995; F. Wolfe, et al. 'Work and disability status of persons with fibromyalgia.' *J Rheumatol* 24:1171–78, 1997; G. O. Littlejohn. 'Fibrositis/fibromyalgia syndrome in the workplace.' *Rheum Dis Clin N Am* 15:45–60, 1989; D. Bruusgaard, et al. 'Fibromyalgia – a new cause for disability pension.' *Scand J Soc Med* 21:116–119, 1993; P. A. Reilly. 'Fibromyalgia in the workplace: A "management" problem.' *Ann Rheum Dis* 52:249–251, 1993; P. A. Reilly. '"Repetitive strain injury": From Australia to the UK.' *J Psychosom Res* 39:783–88, 1996; F. Wolfe, et al. 'Health status and disease severity in fibromyalgia.' *Arthritis Rheum* 40:1571–79, 1997; N. M. Hadler. 'Back pain in the workplace. What you lift or how you lift matters far less than whether you lift or when.' *Spine* 22:935–40, 1997; N. M. Hadler. 'Workers with disabling back pain.' *N Eng J Med* 337:341–43, 1997.

169, 170. For studies regarding managed health care and chronic illness, see A. Trafford. 'The empathy gap.' *The Washington Post* August 29, page 6, 1995; A. J. Barsky and J. F. Borus. 'Somatization and medicalization in the era of managed care.' *JAMA* 274:1931–34, 1995; R. A. Knox. 'The rush is on in doctors' offices.' *The Boston Globe* March 2:1, 1996; M. F. Shore and A. Beigel. 'The challenges posed by managed behavioral health care.' *N Eng J Med* 334:116–118, 1996. The book, T. B. McCall. *Examining Your Doctor: A Patient's Guide to Avoiding Harmful Medical Care,* Secaucus: Carol Publishing Group, 1995, provides practical guidelines for working with your doctor and flags the problems to watch out for.

171. Quote from L. Slater. *Welcome To My Country.* Random House, New York, 1996, pg. 13. This book describes Slater's personal and professional experiences with mental illness.

172, 173. S. H. Kaplan, et al. 'Characteristics of physicians with participatory decision-making styles.' *Ann Intern Med* 124:497–504, 1996.

174, 175. The role of support groups, see E. Neerinckx, B. Van Houdenhove, R. Lysnes, H Vertommen, and P. Onghena. 'Attributions in chronic fatigue syndrome and fibromyalgia syndrome in tertiary care.' *J Rheumatol* 27:1051–1055, 2000. Previous contact with self-help groups had a negative impact on illness attributions. Quote on pg. 174 from the 8 July, 2000 *New York Times* article by David Grann, 'Stalking Doctor Steere,' pg. 57.

CHAPTER 16

177–179. To review the role of education and information in fibromyalgia and rheumatic diseases, see P. M. Nicassio, et al. 'A comparison of behavioral and educational interventions for fibromyalgia.' *J Rheumatol* 24:2000–7, 1997; L. A. Bradley and K. R. Alberts. 'Psychological and behavioral approaches to pain management for patients with rheumatic disease.' *Rheum Dis Clin N Am* 25:215–32, 1998; C. S. Burckhardt and A. Bjelle. 'Education programs for fibromyalgia patients: Description and evaluation.' *Baillieres Clin Rheumatol* 8:935–955, 1994.

179. G. L. Engel. 'The need for a new medical model: A challenge for biomedicine.' *Science* 196:129–36, 1977.

179, 180. Studies of the efficacy of comprehensive treatment programmes in fibromyalgia include: R. M. Bennett, et al. 'Group treatment of fibromyalgia: A 6 month outpatient programme.' *J Rheumatol* 23:521–528, 1996; G. A. McCain. 'A cost-effective approach to the diagnosis and treatment of fibromyalgia.' *Rheum Dis Clin N Am* 22:323–349, 1996; D. L. Goldenberg. 'Management of fibromyalgia syndrome.' *Rheum Dis Clin N Am* 15:499–512, 1989. Quote by Charcot on pg. 178 from H. C. Coghlan. 'Functional syndromes: Are they really functional?' *J Funct Syn* 1:5–13, 2001, pg. 5.

180, 181. Coping strategies and the adverse impact of hopelessness and catastrophizing are discussed in B. C. Kersh, et al. 'Psychosocial and health status variables independently predict health care seeking in fibromyalgia.' *Arthritis Rheum* 45:362–71, 2001; C. S. Burckhardt and A. Bjelle. 'Perceived control: a comparison of women with fibromyalgia, rheumatoid arthritis, and systemic lupus erythematosus using a Swedish version of the Rheumatology Attitudes Index.' *Scand J Rheumatol* 25:300–6, 1996; L. A. Aaron, et al. 'Catastrophizing is a specific moderator of daily pain and health status in patients with fibromyalgia.' *Arthritis Rheum* 40: S129, 1997; C. Henriksson, et al. 'Living with fibromyalgia: Consequences for everyday life.' *Clin J Pain* 8:138–144, 1992. For more discussion of the negative physiological effects of pain anticipation, see M. Lekander, et al. 2000.

181–182. Quote from Dalai Lama and H. C. Cutler. *The Art of Happiness*, New York: Riverhead Books, 1998, pg. 148.

181, 182. Potential adverse effects of blaming physical trauma as the cause of fibromyalgia are discussed in L. A. Aaron, et al. 'Perceived physical and emotional trauma as precipitating events in fibromyalgia. Associations with health care seeking and disability status but not pain severity.' *Arthritis Rheum* 40:453–60, 1997; S. Greenfield, et al. 'Reactive fibromyalgia syndrome.' *Arthritis Rheum* 35:678–681, 1992.

182–183. Quote from Groopman, *The New Yorker* 2000, pg. 90.

183–185. For studies on the prognosis and outcome of fibromyalgia, see F. Wolfe, et al. 'A prospective, longitudinal, multicenter study of service utilization and costs in fibromyalgia.' *Arthritis Rheum* 40:1560–70, 1997; D. H. Solomon and M. H. Liang. 'Fibromyalgia: Scourge of humankind or bane of a rheumatologist's existence?' *Arthritis Rheum* 40:1553–55, 1997; D. T. Felson and D. L. Goldenberg. 'The natural history of fibromyalgia.' *Arthritis Rheum* 29:1522–1526, 1986; G. Granges, et al. 'Fibromyalgia syndrome: assessment of the severity of the condition 2 years after diagnosis.' *J Rheumatol* 21:523–529, 1994; G. S. Alarcon and L. A. Bradley. 'Advances in the treatment of fibromyalgia: current status and future directions.' *Am J Med Sci* 315:397–404, 1998; Two recent reports indicate that the outcome in fibromyalgia is better than had been previously thought: A. M. Mengshoel, et al. 'Health status in fibromyalgia – a follow-up study.' *J Rheumatol* 28:2089–9, 2001. 51 women with fibromyalgia were evaluated 8 years after the diagnosis and there was no overall worsening of their symptoms and no change in their employment status. R. Payhia, et al. 'Pain and pain relief in fibromyalgia patients followed for three years.' *Arthritis Rheum* 45:355–61, 2001. In this study, 82 women with fibromyalgia were evaluated each year for three consecutive years. In general there was a spontaneous improvement in their pain as well as less medication use over time.

EPILOGUE

185. See Weil, *Health and Healing.*

186. From L. Thomas. *The Medusa and the Snail,* New York: Viking, 1979.

186, 187. From H. Mandell and H. Spiro. *When Doctors Get Sick,* New York: Plenum Medical Book Company, 1987, pg. 456.

GLOSSARY

acupressure: see acupuncture; uses pressure rather than needles.

acupuncture: an ancient Eastern healing treatment during which thin needles are inserted at specific meridian points. Said to change energy flow and decrease pain; more accepted now in Western medicine.

adrenaline: hormone that activates the sympathetic nervous system and is important in maintaining body functions such as heart rate and blood pressure.

allodynia: pain from a stimulus that normally does not produce pain.

alternative treatments: also termed 'complementary medicine'; treatment not considered to be part of standard approved drugs or other therapies.

analgesic: any medication that reduces pain.

antinuclear antibody (ANA): blood test used to confirm the diagnosis of lupus, but often positive in people without serious illness.

aura: neurological symptoms, usually including visual changes such as flashing lights or moving lines, typically at the start of a migraine headache.

autonomic nervous system: also called the 'sympathetic nervous system,' an unconscious and automatic area of the nervous system that helps communicate signals to organs such as blood vessels and glands, playing a major role in maintaining blood pressure and heart rates.

benign myalgic encephalomyelitis: term sometimes used interchangably with 'chronic fatigue syndrome.'

benzodiazepines: a class of drugs with sedative properties, often used to treat anxiety and sleep disturbances.

biofeedback: a relaxation technique utilized to decrease muscle tension and sometimes used to change temperature or pain perception.

candidiasis: a yeast infection.

CAT scans: the formal term is 'computerized axial tomography' and refers to imaging studies creating a three-dimensional picture that is more detailed and more accurate than plain X-rays.

caudate nucleus: a part of the brain that is important in pain processing.

celecoxib (Celebrex): one of the newer anti-inflammatory medications, called 'Cox-2 inhibitors,' since they inhibit the second cyclo-oxygenase enzyme and are less likely to cause bleeding than the earlier NSAIDs.

central sensitization: refers to the role of the central nervous system in pain and the fact that the brain and the spinal cord may become super-sensitized to pain, thereby accelerating pain messages.

cerebral cortex: a part of the brain including the cerebral hemispheres (cerebral cortex and basal ganglia).

charlatans: practise medical fraud, claiming to cure disease by useless procedures or worthless diagnostic and therapeutic tests, i.e., quackery.

Chiari syndrome: a congenital displacement and herniation of the base of the brain, said, in rare situations, to contribute to or cause fibromyalgia. This claim is not well substantiated.

chiropractic: a system said to use recuperative powers of the body and adjusting relationships between the musculoskeletal structures and functions of the body to treat various disorders.

citalopram: a serotonin reuptake inhibitor typically used for the treatment of mood disturbances.

classic migraine: migraine headaches accompanied by visual aura and other neurological symptoms.

clonazepam: a benzodiazepine medication often used for the treatment of anxiety and sleep disturbances.

cognitive behavioural: any treatment that utilizes talk therapy or other techniques to modify a person's behaviour that is felt to be damaging to their health.

cognitive disturbances: problems with memory, concentration, or other intellectual activities.

common migraine: migraine headaches that are not associated with aura.

complementary therapies: any form of treatment not mainstream or not traditionally performed by doctors.

corticosteroids: a powerful group of anti-inflammatory medications naturally produced by the adrenal cortex that have an immunosuppressive effect.

corticotrophin-releasing hormone (CRH): a hormone that regulates the release of corticosteroids from the adrenal gland.

costochondritis: inflammation of cartilage in the chest wall.

cytokines: proteins that are important in inflammation and immunity.

disc herniation: a term often used to describe vertebral disc protrusion or bulge that may or may not be the source of back or neck pain.

ecologist: a health-care provider who focuses on inter-relationships among humans and the environment and how these could cause illness.

endorphins: hormones that the body manufactures having a pain relieving effect as powerful as opioids.

Epstein-Barr virus (EBV): the virus that initially was thought to be a possible cause of CFS.

Feldenkrais: a therapy that teaches how the body moves in space.

fentanyl (Durogesic): a long-acting opioid that is worn on a patch.

fibrositis: the old term for fibromyalgia.

fluoxetine (Prozac): a serotonin reuptake inhibitor (SSRI) antidepressant.

gabepentin (Neurontin): an antiseizure medication that has also been used to treat pain and mood disorders.

growth hormone: a natural hormone that is important in body growth and muscle strength.

guaifenesin: a substance found in cough expectorants and claimed by some to help treat fibromyalgia.

herbs: plant-derived substances.

herniated disc: see disc herniation.

homeopathy: a system of therapy, developed by Samuel Hahnemann, based on the 'law of similars,' which holds that a medicinal substance that can evoke certain symptoms in healthy individuals may be effective in the treatment of illnesses if given in very small doses.

hyperalgesia: excessive sensitivity to painful stimuli.

hypothalamic-pituitary-adrenal (HPA) axis: the communication system from the brain to glands that secrete various hormones that are very important in stress and immune responses.

ibuprofen (Brufen, Nurofen): a commonly used NSAID, available on prescription or over the counter.

idiopathic pain: pain of unknown origin.

interleukin: cytokines synthesized by lymphocytes and other cells that are important in inflammation and immunity.

interstitial cystitis: inflammation of the bladder, common in fibromyalgia but overlaps with irritable bladder and with irritable urethral syndrome.

lactic acid: chemical that accumulates in muscle during exercise.

L-Dopa/carbidopa (Sinemet): a drug combination used to treat Parkinson's disease, but also effective treatment for restless leg syndrome.

lidocaine: an anaesthetic usually given by injection.

lorazepam (Ativan): a benzodiazepine used for anxiety and sleep disturbances.

lumbago: archaic name for back pain.

magnetic resonance imaging (MRI): an imaging technique that uses magnetic energy to create very sensitive three-dimensional images of the body and the brain and is more sensitive than plain X-rays with no X-ray exposure.

melatonin: a hormone made in the pineal gland that is important in sleep and skin pigmentation.

morphine: one of the strongest opioid analgesics.

myalgia: muscle pain.

myofascial pain: a more localized form of fibromyalgia, characterized by trigger points and referred pain.

naproxen (Naprosyn, Synflex): one of the first NSAIDs, now available over the counter.

naturopath: provides health care using only natural (non-medicinal) forces.

neurohormones: a hormone secreted by neural cells, such as adrenaline.

neuron: the major cell of the nervous system.

neuroplasticity: the concept that responses, such as pain, can have ever-changing effects.

nociceptors: a peripheral nerve that receives and transmits painful messages.

nonsteroidal anti-inflammatory medications (NSAIDs): medications that work against tissue inflammation, as well as pain, including salicylates, ibuprofen, and naproxen.

noradrenaline: a natural catecholamine that has hormonal effects on the autonomic nervous sysysem that differ from those of adrenaline.

objective: can be proven by unbiased evidence.

opioid: any analgesic structurally derived from opium.

orthostatic hypotension: excessive fall in blood pressure when standing or changing body posture.

osteopaths: their treatment is based on the concept that the body, when in correct adjustment, makes its own remedies.

paraesthesias: numbness and tingling sensations.

paroxetine (Seroxat): a serotonin reuptake inhibitor (SSRI) antidepressant.

Percocet: an analgesic consisting of oxycodone and paracetamol. Not available in the U.K.

phantom limb pain: pain felt to be coming from an extremity that has been amputated.

physiatrist: a physician trained in rehabilitative medicine.

physical therapy: an American term for any treatment using physical techniques, such as moving or stretching or applying ultrasound.

Pilates: a form of exercise and body movement introduced by Joseph Pilates.

placebo: any drug or intervention that creates a non-specific therapeutic effect, not related to the known action or properties of that drug.

prednisone: the commonest corticosteroid used to treat inflammatory diseases.

psychogenic: symptoms coming from the brain that affect functions of the body.

quackery: medical fraud.

Raynaud's phenomenon: vascular spasm of the fingers and toes, usually brought on by cold.

rheumatism: a non-specific term for musculoskeletal aches and pain, which include arthritis as well as fibromyalgia.

rheumatoid arthritis: the most common inflammatory, systemic arthritis, affecting about 1 percent of the population. It is an immunological disorder that, if untreated, can cause joint damage in many parts of body, especially the fingers and toes.

rheumatologist: a physician trained in internal medicine who then specializes in the treatment of arthritis and related conditions.

serotonin: a hormone with vast effects, including on mood, sleep, pain, gastric secretion, and smooth muscle; found in high concentrations in some areas of the central nervous system especially the hypothalamus and basal ganglia. Also referred to as 5-hydroxytryptamine in medical and pharmacological literature.

serotonin reuptake inhibitors (SSRIs): antidepressants that exert some of their effect by blocking the reuptake of serotonin, but also affect other neurohormones.

sicca syndrome: dry eyes and dry mouth, as seen in some normal people, but more common in autoimmune diseases.

slipped disc: see disc herniation.

SPECT scan: an imaging technique that is based on the spectrum of electrical wavelength activity.

spinal stenosis: narrowing in the spinal canal, often due to arthritis or degenerative disc changes, that can lead to weakness and neurological impairment.

subjective: related to personal experience.

subluxations: body parts that are out of alignment; usually refers to vertebrae.

substance P: a substance that is important in pain transmission, especially at nerve endings.

sumatriptan (Imgran): a drug that activates the vascular 5-hydroxytryptamine receptor and was designed specifically to abort the onset of a migraine attack.

systemic lupus erythematosus (lupus): a systemic connective tissue disorder related to the immunological production of various autoantibodies. The name comes from the typical skin rash, but lupus can affect multiple organs.

temporomandibular joint syndrome (TMJ): a syndrome characterized by jaw and facial pains, sometimes felt related to misalignment of the jaw, but, at other times, felt to be a form of myofascial pain syndrome.

tender points: specific sites where muscle attaches to the bone or joint that are excessively tender upon modest pressure.

thalamus: a section of the brain near the internal capsule and the caudate nucleus, which is very important in directing sensory messages throughout the central nervous system.

tramadol (Zydol, Zamadol): a pain reliever that has different analgesic activity than opioids and has some effect on the serotonin system.

tricyclic antidepressants: a large group of antidepressant medications that include amitriptyline; their name is derived from the three-ring structure of the basic chemical compound.

trigger point: a specific site, usually in the muscle, that is tender to pressure and is associated with taut muscle and creates referred pain.

venlaxafine (Effexor): an antidepressant with both serotonin and noradrenaline reuptake activity, sometimes used in fibromyalgia.

rofecoxib (Vioxx): one of the new cyclooxygenase-2 inhibitors used for analgesic and anti-inflammatory conditions.

vulvodynia: idiopathic pelvic pain.

sertraline (Lustral): a serotonin-reuptake inhibitor antidepressant (SSRI).

Zolpidem (Stilnoct): a drug used for sleep disturbances.

ADDITIONAL RESOURCES

BOOKS MENTIONED OR RECOMMENDED

Amand, R. P., Marek, C. C. *What Your Doctor May Not Tell You About Fibromyalgia*. New York: Warner Books, 1999.

Aronowitz, R. *Making Sense of Illness: Science, Society, and Disease*. Cambridge: Cambridge University Press, 1998.

Dubovsky, S. *Mind Body Deceptions: The Psychosomatics of Everyday Life*. New York: W. W. Norton & Company, Inc., 1997.

Fishman, S., Berger, L. *The War on Pain*. New York: HarperCollins Publishers, 2000.

Goldenberg, D. L. *Chronic Illness and Uncertainty: A Personal and Professional Guide to Poorly Understood Syndromes*. Newton, MA: Dorset Press, 1997.

Groopman, J. *Second Opinions*. New York: Penguin Group, Penguin Putnam, Inc., 2000.

Hahn, R. *Sickness and Healing: An Anthropological Perspective*. New Haven: Yale University Press, 1995.

Jamison, K. R. *An Unquiet Mind: A Memoir of Moods and Madness*. New York: Vintage Books, 1995.

Jamison, K. R. *Night Falls Fast: Understanding Suicide*. New York: Alfred A. Knopf, 1999.

Johnson, H. *Osler's Web*. New York: Crown, 1996.

Kabat-Zinn, J. *Full Catastrophe Living: Using Wisdom of Your Body and Mind to Face Stress, Pain, and Illness*. Delacorte Press, 1990.

Kabat-Zinn, J. *Mindfulness Meditation for Everyday Life*. London, Piatkus Books, 1994.

Kleinman, A. *The Illness Narratives: Suffering, Healing and the Human Condition*. Basic Books, 1988.

Dalai Lama, Cutler, H. C. *The Art of Happiness*. New York: Riverhead Books, 1998.

Mandell, H., Spiro, H. *When Doctors Get Sick*. New York: Plenum Medical Book Company, 1987.

Mayou, R., Bass, C. M., Sharpe M. *Treatment of Functional Somatic Symptoms*. New York: Oxford University Press, 1995.

McCall, T. B. *Examining Your Doctor: A Patient's Guide to Avoiding Harmful Medical Care*. Secaucus: Carol Publishing Group, 1995.

Micale, M. *Approaching Hysteria: Disease and Its Interpretations*. Princeton: Princeton University Press, 1995.

Nelson, D. *Selling Science, Revised Edition: How the Press Covers Science and Technology*. New York: W. H. Freeman and Company, 1995.

Sacks, O. *Migraine: Revised and Expanded*. Berkeley: University of California Press, 1992.

Salt II, W. B. *Irritable Bowel Syndrome & the Mind-Body Brain-Gut Connection*. Columbus: Parkview Publishing, 1997.

Sarno, J. E. *The Mindbody Prescription: Healing the Body, Healing the Pain*. New York: Warner Books, 1998.

Shapiro, A, Shapiro, E. *The Powerful Placebo: From Ancient Priest to Modern Physician*. Baltimore: The Johns Hopkins University Press, 1997.

Shorter, E. *From Paralysis to Fatigue: A History of Psychosomatic Illness in the Modern Era*. New York: The Free Press, 1992.

Shorter, E. *A History of Psychiatry*. New York: John Wiley & Sons, Inc., 1997.

Showalter, E. *Hystories: Hysterical Epidemics and Modern Media*. New York: Columbia University Press, 1997.

Slater, L. *Welcome to My Country*. New York: Random House, 1996.

Spiro, H. *The Power of Hope: A Doctor's Perspective*. New Haven: Yale University Press, 1998.

Weil, A. *Health and Healing*. Time Warner Paperbacks, 1996.

Wheelwright, J. *The Irritable Heart*. New York: W. W. Norton, 2001.

WEB SITES MENTIONED OR RECOMMENDED

Fibromyalgia and musculoskeletal disorders

The American College of Rheumatology: http://www.rheumatology.org

The Arthritis Foundation: http://www.arthritis.org

U.K. Local Support: http://www.ostrust.freeserve.co.uk/self-help.htm

The Oregon Fibromyalgia Foundation: http://www.myalgia.com

Fibromyalgia Network: http://www.fmnetnews.com

Fibromyalgia Association U.K.: http://www.fmsni.freeserve.co.uk/fmauk.htm

National Fibromyalgia Partnership, Inc.: http://www.fmpartnership.org

Fibromyalgia Association of Greater Washington: http://www.fmagw.org

British Columbia Fibromyalgia Association: http://www.alternatives.com/bcfms

Related illnesses

American Association for CFS: http://www.aacfs.org

Irritable Bowel Syndrome Association: http://www.ibsassociation.org

Migraine site: http://www.ama-assn.org/special/migraine

Other helpful sites

National Center for Complementary and Alternative Medicine: http://nccam.nih.gov/

The American Pain Society: http://www.AmPainSoc.org

The Partners Against Pain: http://www.PartnersAgainstPain.com

The Pain and Policy Studies Group site hosted by University of Wisconsin: http://www.medsch.wisc.edu/painpolicy

British Chiropractic Association: http://www.chiropractic-uk.co.uk

For herbs, see: HerbMed http://www.herbmed.org/

FDA Dietary Supplements, see http://www.cfsan.fda.gov/~dms/supplmnt.html

MedWatch (The FDA medical reporting system): http://www.fda.gov/medwatch/

CDC Web site: http://www.cdc.gov/

Mayo Clinic: http://www.mayoclinic.com

Feldenkrais: http://www.feldenkrais-resources.com

National Institute of Medical Herbalists: http://www.nimh.org.uk

Pilates Web sites: http://www.pilatesfoundation.com/

INDEX

Page numbers in *italic* indicate figures; those in **bold** indicate tables.